**Biblical Foundations for Divine Healing**

By Larry L Yates ThD, DMin

ISBN: 978-1-52019-994-8

Copyright© 2019 by Miracles in Action/Larry L Yates

Unless otherwise noted all Scripture quotations in this book are from the King James Version of the Bible

Printed in the United States

Printed by Miracles in Action

## Dedication

To the memory of John G. Lake, the Apostle to Africa and to the example he left us of how to walk in the righteousness, authority and dominion that is ours as Children of God.

"And Jesus went about all Galilee, teaching in their synagogues, and preaching the gospel of the kingdom, and healing all manner of sickness and all manner of disease among the people."

--Matthew 4:23

"Then He called His twelve disciples together, and gave them power and authority over all devils, and to cure diseases. And He sent them to preach the Kingdom of God, and heal the sick."

--Luke 9:1, 2

"And these signs shall follow them that believe; in my Name…they shall lay hands on the sick and they shall recover."

--Mark 16:17, 18

☐

# Contents

# CHAPTER 1

## THE WORD OF GOD IS OUR ULTIMATE RULE OF FAITH AND ACTION

### The Word of God: A More Sure Covenant

The Word is our final authority. Our experiences must be judged by Scripture not Scripture judged by experiences.

The Word of God is forever settled in Heaven, we must settle it on earth.

*Psalms 119:89-92 (KJV) 89. Forever, O Lord, thy word is settled in heaven. 90. Thy faithfulness is unto all generations: thou hast established the earth, and it abideth. 91. They continue this day according to thine ordinances: for all are thy servants. 92. Unless thy law had been my delights, I should then have perished in mine affliction.*

*Hebrews 8:6 (KJV) But now hath he obtained a more excellent ministry, by how much also He is the mediator of a better covenant, which was established upon better promises.*

The Word of God is unchanging, unmoving. What it says today, it will say 100 years from now. You should believe it today. Don't wait 20 years; it will still be the same.

We settle God's Word on earth by believing in it, standing on it, fighting for it, receiving it.

A "Will" reveals the nature and intentions of the person who wrote it.

The Sovereignty of God is not the fickleness of God. The Sovereignty of God cannot mean that He has the right to pick and choose whom He will keep His word to. If that were true, we could never pray the prayer of faith as commanded in James 5:14-16.

**You cannot have faith any further than your knowledge of what the will of God is.**

NOTE: There is no such thing in the Bible as an "unspoken request". An unspoken request is an unanswered request. Before you can agree with someone in prayer about something, you must know what it is.

**The written Word of God is more sure than a voice speaking from Heaven.**

*2 Peter 1:16-21 16. For we have not followed cunningly devised fables, when we made known unto you the power and coming of our Lord Jesus Christ, but were eyewitnesses of His majesty. 17. For we received from God the Father honor and glory, when there came such a voice to him from the excellent glory, "This is my beloved Son, In whom I am well pleased". 18. And this voice, which came from heaven, we heard, when we were with him in the holy mount. 19. We have also a more sure word of prophecy; whereunto ye do well that ye take heed, as unto a light that shines in a dark place, until the day dawn, and the day star arise in your hearts: 20. Knowing this first, that no prophecy of the scripture is of any private interpretation. 21. For the prophecy came not in old time by the will of man: but holy men of God spoke as the Holy Ghost moved them. (KJV)*

Once We Accept the Word of God As Our Final Authority, We Must Begin To Retrain Our Mind To Think In Line With God's Will

The Bible is the revealed will of God. Everything that we need to know about how to live the way God wants us to, must be, and has been provided to us.

God cannot require you to do what you cannot do.

God cannot hold you responsible for what you cannot know.

*Romans. 12: 1-2 – 1. I beseech you therefore, brethren, by the mercies of God, that ye present your bodies a living sacrifice, holy, acceptable unto God, which is your reasonable service. 2. And be not conformed to this world: but be ye transformed by the renewing of your mind, that ye may prove what is the good, and acceptable, and perfect, will of God.*

God requires us to "prove" what is the good, acceptable, and perfect will of God. If God's will changes from minute to minute and from person to person, we can never, with certainty, know, let alone prove His will.

This brings us to the question of how to prove what God's will is. This question is answered in the same verse that commands us to prove it. *".... But ye be transformed by the renewing of your mind..."*

You must renew your mind by the Word of God. You renew your mind by changing the way you think about things, until every thought agrees with what the Bible says about it. To do this you must:

Systematically study the Bible to find out what it says about each topic.

Form what you learn into a statement (often called a confession) that helps you remember the biblical position.

Since your mind works like a computer, whatever is in your memory will stay there until it is deleted and replaced with new information. Because of this, it is not enough to learn Bible Scriptures; you must pull down any thought that does not agree with the Bible.

*1 Corinthians. 10:3-5 (KJV) – 3. For though we walk in the flesh, we do not war after the flesh. 4. For the weapons of our warfare are not carnal, but mighty through God to the pulling down of strongholds. 5. Casting down imaginations, and every high thing that exalted itself against the knowledge of God, and bringing into captivity every thought to the obedience of Christ.*

For the Word of God to be truly effective in our lives, we must reach and live in a place where our first thought is what the Bible says. Not "what does the Bible say", but rather we think in line with the Word, when this occurs we are experiencing our Biblical positional standing in Christ as one who has the mind of Christ.

*1 Corinthians. 2: 12-16* – *12. Now we have received, not the spirit of the world, but the spirit, which is of God; that we might know the things that are freely given to us of God. 13. Which things also we speak, not in the words which man's wisdom teaches, but which the Holy Ghost teaches; comparing spiritual things with spiritual. 14. But the natural man receiveth not the things of the Spirit of God: for they are foolishness unto him: neither can he know them, because they are spiritually discerned. 15. But he that is spiritual judges all things, yet he himself is judged of no man. 16. For who hath known the mind of the Lord, that he may instruct Him? But we have the mind of Christ. (KJV)*

*Ephesians. 4: 22-24* – 22. *That ye put off the former conversation of the old man, which is corrupt according to the deceitful lusts. 23. And be renewed in the spirit of your mind; 24. And that ye put on the new man, which after God is created in righteousness and true holiness. (KJV)*

*Col. 3: 10-11* – *And have put on the new man, which is renewed in knowledge after the image of him that created him: Where there is neither Greek nor Jew, circumcision nor uncircumcision, Barbarian, Scythian, bond nor free: but Christ is all, and in all. (KJV)*

When we are born into the Kingdom of God, we are born into the royal family; all rights of royalty are already there. Yet still we do not exercise our rights to dominion in every possible area because of our limited knowledge and understanding of those rights. As we learn of our rights and responsibilities as the children of God, (by having our minds renewed to line up with the Word of God) we begin to look more and more like our elder brother Jesus.

This "renewing" is what allows what is inside us to come out. To fully allow the "real" you to come forth, you must know what the Word of God has to say about every subject AND you must begin to ACT on every scripture that you learn.

**Finally, let's look at something that is probably more important in the area of healing than in any other area.**

*Romans. 8:14* - *For as many as are led by the Spirit of God, they are the sons of God. (KJV)*

*James 1:22* - *But be ye doers of the word, and not hearers only, deceiving your own selves. (KJV)*

Based upon the current teaching prevalent in the church, many would say that these two verses are contradictory. The way Romans 8:14 is usually used is to promote the idea that a Christian is not supposed to do anything that they are not "led by the Spirit" to do.

There are those that try to say that Christians should only do something when they receive a *"Rhema"* word from God.

First, let me say that they should go back and read all of Romans 8 and put verse 14 in context. The context there has nothing to do with a Christian "doing" anything other than

16

mortifying the deeds of the flesh. It especially does NOT say that a Christian should not exercise any of the benefits of the Atonement, or that they should not obey any and every Scripture that can apply to them.

If it did, we would have to add, "if the Spirit leads you to" before every command in the New Testament.

This would also make James 1:22 not only misleading, but it would make God guilty of making you sin. Because, how are you supposed to know when to act on a Scripture and when not to act on a Scripture.

Your mission, as a Christian, is to manifest the Lord Jesus Christ in each and every situation that you are involved in.

You are anointed by God.

*1 John 2:27* - *But the anointing in which ye have received of him abides in you, and ye need not that any man teach you: but as the same anointing teaches you of all things, and is truth, and is no lie, and even as it hath taught you, ye shall abide in him. (KJV)*

A child of God is destined to be conformed to the image of Christ.

**Romans. 8:29** - *For whom he did foreknow, he also did predestinate to be conformed to the image of His Son, that he might be the firstborn among many brethren. (KJV)*

You are commissioned to do the works that Jesus did and greater works than He did BECAUSE He went to the Father. (He did His part by going, now it's our turn and our job is to do the greater works).

**John 14:12-14** – *12. Verily, verily, I say unto you, He that believeth on me, the works that I do shall he do also; and greater works than these shall he do; because I go unto my Father. 13. And whatsoever ye shall ask in my name, that will I do, that the Father may be glorified in the Son. 14. If ye shall ask anything in my name, I will do it. (KJV)*

You are sent as He was sent.

**John 20:21** - *Then said Jesus to them again, Peace be unto you: as my Father hath sent me, even so I send you.*

You are to do the same thing He did, which was:

*1 John 3:8* - *He that committeth sin is of the devil; for the devil hath sinned from the beginning. For this purpose the Son of God was manifested, that he might destroy the works of the devil.*

How did Jesus destroy the works of the devil?

*Acts 10:38* - *God anointed Jesus of Nazareth with the Holy Ghost and with power: who went about doing good, and healing all that were oppressed of the devil, for God was with Him. (KJV)*

## AND THAT'S HOW YOU WILL DO IT TOO!

# CHAPTER 2

## THE DIVINE HEALING COVENANT

God always begins a relationship (with a person or with a nation) by revealing His Name, (just as we do), which in turn reveals His Nature and His Attitude toward them.

*Exodus. 3:13-14 – And Moses said unto God, Behold, when I come unto the children of Israel, and shall say unto them, The God of your fathers hath sent me unto you; and they shall say unto me, what is his name? What shall I say unto them? 14. And God said unto Moses, I AM THAT I AM: and he said, Thus shall thou say unto the children of Israel, I AM hath sent me unto you. (KJV)*

God's name is "I AM" – This signifies the truth that God is the God who always IS. He is not the God Who Was, or the God Who Shall Be, He is the God Who Is.

God is always NOW, which is why faith is always Now (Hebrews 11:1) (If it's not now, it's not faith it's hope)

God is not constantly changing. He is always the same.

**Malachi 3:6** – *For I am the Lord, I change Not…. (KJV)*

We are still dealing with the same God today that Abraham dealt with.

There has been no shift change. You are not dealing with an employee but with THE OWNER.

**The divine order or procedure of revelation or the revealing of things to man, has, is, and always will be, line upon line, precept upon precept, here a little, there a little.**

*Isaiah. 28: 9-10 – Whom shall he teach knowledge? And whom shall he make to understand doctrine? Them that are weaned from the milk, and drawn from the breasts. 10. For precept must be upon precept, precept upon precept, line upon line, here a little, there a little: (KJV)*

The divine procedure is to reveal truth little by little. Thus giving man the time and opportunity to grow into the knowledge he is gaining. The important thing to remember is that each

22

successive revelation builds upon the previous revelation rather than destroying it to start over.

Jesus said in

**Matthew 5:17-19** – *Think not that I have come to destroy the law, or the prophets: I have not come to destroy, but to fulfill. 18. For verily I say unto you, till heaven and earth pass, one jot or one tittle shall in no wise pass from the law, till all be fulfilled. 19. Whosoever therefore shall break one of these least commandments, and shall teach men so, he shall be called the least in the kingdom of heaven: but whosoever shall do and teach them, the same shall be called great in the kingdom of heaven.*

Each new bit of information we get from The Word of God should be added to our understanding to allow us a clearer picture of the God we serve.

**The first revelation we have is that Whatever God is, He Always IS. Remember that in the Bible, names always meant something; they described the thing they were attached to.**

Abraham- Father of Many Nations

Jacob- Usurper/Deceiver- who became Israel which means "Prince with God".

**When God gives us a name by which He desires to be called by us, He is telling us Who He wants to be to us. Bible scholars say that God has given to man a series of what are called "covenant" or "redemptive" names, which are names by which God has made covenants or unbreakable contracts with mankind. One of these names is found in Exodus.**

*Exodus 15:26* - *"...if thou wilt diligently hearken to the voice of the Lord thy God, and wilt do that which is right in his sight, and wilt give ear to his commandments, and keep all his statutes, I will put none of these diseases upon thee, which I have brought upon the Egyptians: for I am the Lord that healeth thee."*

When this verse is read in the original Hebrew, the last part of the verse, which reads; "for I am the Lord that healeth thee.", is actually a name: *"Jehovah-Rapha"*. Once God established the name Jehovah-Rapha as a name that applied to Him, He revealed to man that he is a God that will forever be man's healer, if man will meet the conditions set down by God.

The conditions of Jehovah-Rapha:

- *if thou wilt diligently hearken to the voice of the Lord thy God,*

- *and wilt do that which is right in His sight,*

- *and wilt give ear to His commandments,*

- *and keep all His statutes,*

The blessings of Jehovah-Rapha

- *I will put none of these diseases upon thee*

- *I AM THE LORD THAT HEALETH THEE*

Many debates have raged over whether God put, caused, brought, or allowed the diseases just mentioned, and if He can and/or will do the same to us today.

The first thing to remember is that He is God, He can and will do whatever is right in His sight, and what is right in His sight IS RIGHT.

The second thing to consider is that the diseases He mentions were put upon the Egyptians, not upon His people. (The Egyptians were the people that had afflicted the Israelites. We must not forget the Law of Sowing and Reaping.)

There is not one verse of Scripture that even suggests that God has ever afflicted one person that was living right before Him.

Objection #1: Job.

Answer: God did not afflict Job, Satan did.

Objection #2: God gave Satan permission.

Answer: Isn't it comforting to know that Satan can do nothing without God's knowledge and permission. Therefore if Satan is attacking us, we know that God is involved.

We know the Bible says the steps of a righteous man are ordered of the Lord, and that, man makes his plans but God directs his steps.

We know that the Bible says "*Thanks be unto God which ALWAYS causes us to triumph IN Christ Jesus*". *(2 Cor. 2:14).*

So what is the conclusion that we must come to if we know that all these things are so? We know this:

Any attack is from Satan

God must give Satan permission before he could attack

If God always makes us win, and we are in the middle of a battle, God, knowing us better than we know ourselves, must know that we have the ability to win this level of warfare, or He would not allow us to be there.

If we are there, we are there to win.

Rejoice when you find that your battles are getting bigger and bigger, it means you are growing. It means Satan is having to send bigger demons to try to stop you.

God, being the Law-giver, the Righteous Judge, and the originator of the Law of Sowing and Reaping, takes the responsibility for the affliction of those who are in sin. In this sense does God send affliction, sickness and disease, etc.? But we also see in Lamentations 3:31-34 that God does not willing afflict. Imagine a man or woman backing God into a corner to where He has to afflict to remain Just and Righteous.

*Lamentations 3:31-33 – 31. For the Lord will not cast off forever: 32. But though he causes grief, yet will he have compassion according to the multitude of his mercies. 33. For he does not afflict willing nor grieve the children of men. (KJV)*

So the first thing to do when, affliction, sickness, disease, etc. come is to judge yourself to make sure all sin is under the blood. During the Lord's Supper or Communion, is a good time to judge yourself. Once you have made sure there is nothing between you that would hinder healing, then you should turn on Satan with the authority of God and command relief. You should not stop or slack up until you EXPERIENCE the desired result. Remember, God is not your problem. He desires that you walk holy and righteously before Him. But if you should miss it and sin, repent before Satan has time to get to God with your sin. No one has a right to change the name of God. If God,

28

in His infinite wisdom knew beforehand all the excesses, all the excuses, all the abuses that man would bring against the name of Jehovah-Rapha, our GOD THAT IS OUR HEALER, and still decided to give us that name to run to in time of need then we would be fools not to take advantage of such wonderful provision.

**Proverbs. 18:10** - *The name of the Lord is a strong tower: the righteous runneth into it, and is safe.*

In the following verse you will notice that one of the conditions of long life, salvation, deliverance, and answered prayer is that we know His Name.

**Psalm 91:14-16** – *14. Because He hath set His love upon me, therefore will I deliver him: I will set him on high, because he hath known my name. 15. He shall call upon me, and I will answer him: I will be with him in trouble; I will deliver him, and honour him. 16. With long life will I satisfy him, and show him my salvation.*

As partakers of a covenant of healing with the great Healer, we should move beyond getting sick and getting well, getting sick and getting well, over and over. We, as children of the

Most High, should realize that if God promises to heal every sickness and disease, and promises that no diseases shall be upon us, then we should live in divine health.

Constant and abiding health that flows from our relationship with God. A health that is the very life of God flowing through our bodies, quickening us and making us alive to the most extreme degree. How can we expect to remain sick or diseased and still fulfill the basic requirement of being a believer that is to lay hands upon the sick and see them healed? (Mark 16:15-20) Man can only give what he has received from God. If he is to represent eternal life, he must at least exhibit a healthy temporal life. This is not to say that if a person is sick, they are not a Christian, it just means that they have not "known His name", so they are not able to partake of the blessing that was so costly for Jesus to obtain, yet so freely offered. Partake of the divine healing covenant today, by covenanting with God that as Jesus died for you, you will live, fully live, for Him.

□

# CHAPTER 3

## DIVINE HEALING IN THE ATONEMENT

**Sin and Sickness are two fruits from The same tree.**

Sin and sickness are always grouped together.

*Psalms 103:2-6* - *2. Bless the LORD, O my soul, and forget not all his benefits: 3. Who forgiveth all thine iniquities; who healeth all thy diseases; 4. Who redeemeth thy life from destruction; who crowneth thee with lovingkindness and tender mercies; 5. Who satisfieth thy mouth with good things; so that thy youth is renewed like the eagle's. 6. The LORD executeth righteousness and judgment for all that are oppressed. (KJV)*

*James 5:13-20* - *13. Is any among you afflicted? Let him pray. Is any merry? Let him sing psalms.14. Is any sick among you? Let him call for the elders of the church; and let them pray over him, anointing him with oil in the name of the Lord: 15. And the prayer of faith shall save the sick, and the Lord shall raise him up; and if he have committed sins, they shall be forgiven him. 16. Confess your faults one to another, and pray one for another, that ye may be healed. The effectual fervent prayer of a righteous man availeth much. 17. Elias was a man subject to like passions as we are, and he prayed earnestly that it might not rain: and it rained not on the earth by the space of three years and six months. 18. And he prayed again, and the heaven gave rain, and the earth brought forth her fruit. 19. Brethren, if any of you do err from the truth, and one convert him; 20. Let him know, that he which converteth the sinner from the error of his way shall save a soul from death, and shall hide a multitude of sins.*

Shall (Strong's #4982 – *sozo*) a soul from death, and shall hide a multitude of sins. (KJV)

Strong's #266 *hamartia* (ham – ar – tee' – ah); a sin. (KJV) – offence, sin (-ful).

i. To miss the mark, to err, be mistaken, to miss or wander from the path of uprightness and honor, to do or go wrong to wander from the law of God, to violate Gods law, to sin.

ii. That which is done wrong, sin, an offense, a violation of divine law in thought or in action.

Strong's #4982 – *sozo* (sode'-zo); Strongs & Thayers – "safe"; to save, i.e. deliver or protect: KJV – heal, preserve, save (self), do well, be (make) whole, to save, to keep safe and sound, to rescue from danger or destruction, from injury or peril, to save a suffering one, (from perishing), that is, one suffering from disease, to make well, to heal, restore to health, to preserve one from danger of destruction, to save or rescue, to save in the biblical sense;

**Sin came into the world by man's (Adam's) sin. (Gen. 3:1-6)**

**Rom. 5:12** - *Wherefore, as by one man sin entered into the world, and death by sin; and so death passed upon all men, for that all have sinned: (KJV)*

**Rom 5:17** - *Fore if by one man's offense death reigned by one; much more they which receive abundance of grace and of the gift of righteousness shall reign in life by one, Jesus Christ. (See also Rom. 5:19-21)*

**Jesus Treated Sin And Sickness The Same. He Removed Them.**

Sickness/Disease

*Matt 9:1-8* – *1. And he entered into a ship, and passed over, and came into his own city. 2. And, behold, they brought to him a man sick of the palsy, lying on a bed: and Jesus seeing their faith said unto the sick of the palsy; Son, be of good cheer; thy sins be forgiven thee. 3. And, behold, certain of the scribes said within themselves, This man blasphemeth. 4.And Jesus knowing their thoughts said, Wherefore think ye evil in your hearts? 5. For whether is easier, to say, Thy sins be forgiven thee; or to say, Arise, and walk? 6. But that ye may know that the Son of man hath power on earth to forgive sins, (then saith he to the sick of the palsy,) Arise, take up thy bed, and go unto thine house.7. And he arose, and departed to his house. 8. But when the multitudes saw it, they marvelled, and glorified God, which had given such power unto men. (KJV)* (See also in Mark 2:1-12 and Luke 5: 17-26)

Sin

*Luke 7:48-50* – *48. And he said unto her, Thy sins are forgiven. 49. And they that sat at meat with him began to say within themselves, Who is this that forgiveth sins also? 50. And he said to the woman, Thy faith hath saved thee; go in peace.*

## Is Healing In The Atonement?

*John 3:14-17* – *14. And as Moses lifted up the serpent in the wilderness, even so must the Son of man be lifted up: 15. That whosoever believeth in him should not perish, but have eternal life. 16. For God so loved the world, that he gave his only begotten Son, that whosoever believeth in him should not perish, but have everlasting life. 17. For God sent not his Son into the world to condemn the world; but that the world through him might be saved.*

*Num 21:4-9* – *4. And they journeyed from mount Hor by the way of the Red sea, to compass the land of Edom: and the soul of the people was much discouraged because of the way. 5. And the people spake against God, and against Moses, Wherefore have ye brought us up out of Egypt to die in the wilderness? for there is no bread, neither is there any water; and our soul loatheth this light bread. 6. And the LORD sent fiery serpents among the people, and they bit the people; and much people of Israel died. 7. Therefore the people came to Moses, and said, We have sinned, for we have spoken against the LORD, and against thee; pray unto the LORD, that he take away the serpents from us. And Moses prayed for the people. 8. And the LORD said unto Moses, Make thee a fiery serpent, and set it upon a pole: and it shall come to pass, that every one that is bitten, when he looketh upon it, shall live.9.And Moses made a serpent of brass, and put it upon a pole, and it came to pass, that if a serpent had bitten any man, when he beheld the serpent of brass, he lived. (KJV)*

Are these two passages referring to the same event?

Answer: Yes.

If this is so, we have a stronger scriptural right to preach healing through Jesus' crucifixion than we do to preach salvation (in its common usage of only eternal life).

The truth is in the preaching and understanding of the "Whole or Full Gospel", that God desires to save man from anything and everything that causes sin, sickness, destruction, or death. This proves that "eternal life" consists of more than just "going to heaven".

**John 10:10** - *"The thief cometh not, but for to steal, and to kill, and to destroy: I have come that they might have life, and that they might have it more abundantly."*

36

*Isaiah. 53:5 - But He was wounded for our transgressions, he was bruised for our iniquities: the chastisement of our peace was upon Him; and with His stripes we are healed.*

*1 Peter 2:24 - Who his own self bare our sins in his body on the tree, that we, being dead to sins, should live unto righteousness: by whose stripes ye are healed.*

The verse here quoted by Peter was originally prophesied by the Prophet Isaiah concerning the Messiah.

The words used for "healed" each time was a word that was only used for physical healing. This was by no mere chance.

These words exactly portray the intent. In Hebrew it was: **Rapha'** (raw-faw'); Strongs#7495 (as in *Jehovah-Rapha*) or raphah; a primitive root; properly, to mend (by stitching), i.e. (figuratively) to cure: KJV cure, (cause to) heal, physician, repair, X thoroughly, make whole.

Always used in reference to physical healing except once- there used in ref. To repairing the temple alter. In Greek it was: *Iaomai* (ee-ah'-om-ahee); Strong's #2390

How do we know that these two verses were referring to the same thing?

Because of **Matt. 8:16-17** – *16. When the even was come, they brought unto him many that were possessed with devils: and he cast out the spirits with his word, and healed all that were sick:17. That it might be fulfilled which was spoken by Esaias the prophet, saying, Himself took our infirmities, and bare our sicknesses. (KJV)*

Some have tried to say that since Jesus "fulfilled" this prophecy He is no longer healing the sick. To follow the same reasoning would force us to say that since Jesus saved those who were following Him at the time He went to the cross, He is no longer saving anyone.

**If Healing is in the Atonement, it is an established fact, it is already DONE.**

Example: If a person puts up a deposit, the deposit is good for as long as the person that put it up wants it to be good.

Jesus made a deposit in His Name, we can draw from that deposit by using His name.

God has made us a standing offer of forgiveness AND healing through the crucifixion.

*Isaiah 53:4* - *Surely He hath borne our griefs, and carried our sorrows: yet we did esteem Him stricken, smitten of God, and afflicted. (KJV)*

Here we see once again the joining of the Atonement with healing of physical sickness.

This is why 1 Peter 2:24 is in the past tense. The deposit or pre-payment for your healing Has been made. "…by whose stripes ye WERE HEALED."

As far as God is concerned, you have been healed; therefore you ARE healed, So act like it. Healing is again connected to the Atonement in Scriptures concerning the "Lord's Supper" or "Communion" in 1 Cor. 11:23-31.

*1 Cor 11:23-31* – *23. For I have received of the Lord that which also I delivered unto you, That the Lord Jesus the same night in which he was betrayed took bread: 24. And when he had given thanks, he broke it, and said, Take, eat: this is my body, which is broken for you: this do in remembrance of me.* (Note that Jesus broke bread first just as He was scourged before He died.) *25. After the same manner also he took the cup, when he had supped, saying, This cup is the new testament in my blood: this do ye, as oft as ye drink it, in remembrance of me. 26. For as often as ye eat this bread, and drink this cup, ye do shew the Lord's death till he come.* (Note that the two are once again found and bound together) *27. Wherefore whosoever shall eat this bread, and drink this cup of the Lord, unworthily, shall be guilty of the body and blood of the Lord. 28. But let a man examine himself, and so let him eat of that bread, and drink of that cup. 29. For he that eateth and drinketh unworthily, eateth and drinketh damnation to himself, not discerning the Lord's body.* (Notice it does not say "the Lord's blood") *30. For this cause many are weak and sickly among you, and many sleep. 31. For if we would judge ourselves, we should not be judged. (KJV)*

(Note that many among you (in the church) are weak, sickly, and some are even asleep in the Lord because they did not discern the Lord's body (not the Lord's blood, but His body). If one can become sick by partaking communion wrongly, then naturally one can obtain healing by partaking correctly.

# CHAPTER 4

## DIVINE HEALING AND THE WILL OF GOD

**What is God's Will?**

*John 10:10*- *The thief cometh not, but for to steal, and to kill, and to destroy: I am come that they might have life, and that they might have it more abundantly. God's will must be that everyone might have life and have it more abundantly.*

*1John 3:8* - *He that committeth sin is of the devil; for the devil sinneth from the beginning. For this purpose the Son of God was manifested, that he might destroy the works of the devil. God's will must be that the works of the devil be destroyed.*

*Acts 10:38* - *How God anointed Jesus of Nazareth with the Hoy Ghost and with power: who went about doing good, and healing all that were oppressed of the devil; for God was with him. God's will must be that if God is with someone, that they should be anointed with the Holy Ghost and with power and* that they go about doing good and healing all that are oppressed of the devil.

*3 Jn. 2* - Beloved, I wish above all things that thou mayest prosper and be in health, even as thy soul prospereth. (KJV)

God's will must be that we prosper and be in health AS our soul prospers.

(Before you can be in health you may have to be healed.)

*Matt. 6: 9, 10* - After this manner therefore pray ye: Our Father which art in heaven, Hallowed be thy name. Thy kingdom come. Thy will be done on earth, as it is in heaven.

God's will must be that His will be done on earth as it is in heaven.

*James 1:22* - But be ye doers of the word, and not hearers only, deceiving your own selves.

God's will must be that we be doers of the Word of God and not just hearers.

There is no qualification as to which "word" we are to be doers of and which "word" we are to ignore.

## What is God's will?

*Matt 22:35-40* – *Then one of them, which was a lawyer, asked him a question, tempting him, and saying, 36. Master, which is the great commandment in the law? 37. Jesus said unto him, Thou shalt love the Lord thy God with all thy heart, and with all thy soul, and with all thy mind. 38. This is the first and great commandment. 39. And the second is like unto it, Thou shalt love thy neighbour as thyself. 40. On these two commandments hang all the law and the prophets.*

## What is God's will?

*Matt. 7:12* - *Therefore all things whatsoever ye should want men to do unto you, do ye even so unto them: for this is the law and the prophets. (KJV)*

If you were sick and someone had the power of God in their life to heal you, would you want them to come to you and minister healing? Anyone who will answer honestly would have to say they would. (In your answer is the commission to the healing ministry!!!)

## Rhema and Logos

In the Greek New Testament there are two primary words translated into English in the KJV as "word":

One of these is #3056 *logos* (log'-os); from 3004; something said (including the thought); by implication a topic (subject of discourse), also reasoning (the mental faculty) or motive; by extension, a computation

The other is #4487 *rhema* (hray'-mah) from #4483; an utterance (individually, collectively or specifically); by implication, a matter or topic (especially of narration, command or dispute); with a negative naught whatever:

As you can tell, there is practically no difference between the two words in the Strong's Concordance Dictionary.

In today's Christianity, we have a teaching that has infected virtually every aspect of the Christian life and doctrine.

We have had "Bible Teachers" tell us that the word *"rhema"* means a special divine impartation or leading. "They" have said that a *Rhema* word from God was necessary before you could act on a Scripture.

They have taught that you do not have to obey or perform every Scripture, just those that the Holy Spirit "quickens" to you.

These "Teachers" must have received a *"rhema"* word from God to get this teaching because it is not in the Bible.

There has been much said about the difference between the two words, *Logos* and *Rhema*. Below is the article reproduced from Vine's Expository Dictionary of Biblical Words.

"The significance of *rhema* (as distinct from *logos*) is exemplified in the injunction to take *"the sword of the Spirit, which is the word of God."* (Eph.6:17). Here the reference is not to the whole Bible as such. But to the individual scripture which the Spirit brings to our remembrance for use in the time of need, a prerequisite being the regular storing of the mind with Scripture. "(Copyright ©1985, Thomas Nelson Publishers)

**Mark 4:14** - *The sower soweth the word (#3056 logos)*

*Mark 16:20* - *And they went forth, and preached every where, the Lord working with them, and confirming the word (#3056 logos) with signs following. Amen.*

*Luke 11:28* - *But he said, Yea rather, blessed are they that hear the word (#3056 logos) of God, and keep it.*

*Rom. 10:17* - *So then faith cometh by hearing, and hearing by the word (#4487 rhema) of God.*

*James 1:22* - *But be ye doers of the word (#3056 logos), and not hearers only, deceiving your own selves.*

**A *"Rhema"* word is any *"Logos"* word that you act upon.**

When you read a scripture you are reading *Logos*, but when you remember that scripture and act upon it in any situation, it becomes *Rhema*.

If you want more *Rhema* start acting upon more *Logos*.

*Matt. 7:24-27* – *24. Therefore whosoever heareth these sayings of mine, and doeth them, I will liken him unto a wise man, which built his house upon a rock: 25. And the rain descended, and the floods came, and the winds blew, and beat upon that house; and it fell not: for it was founded upon a rock. 26. And every one that heareth these sayings of mine, and doeth them not, shall be likened unto a foolish man, which built his house upon the sand: 27. And the rain descended, and the floods came, and the winds blew, and beat upon that house; and it fell: and great was the fall of it.*

What is the purpose or meaning of this story?

Obviously it is to convince us to hear (read) what Jesus has said and is saying AND DO WHAT HE HAS SAID. The only difference between the wise man and the fool is that one did what he heard and one didn't. There is absolutely no indication that any further leading (by the Holy Spirit) or revelation is necessary for one to be responsible to do what he has heard from the Scriptures.

It is always God's will for us to apply (by doing) a Scripture to a situation that the Scriptures can be applied to.

If Jesus is the full expression of God, then why did Jesus NEVER put sickness on even one person? Why did he always remove sickness and disease, rather than put it upon anyone?

Jesus had "healing services" every day, NOT ONCE did He EVER tell anyone to keep their sickness or disease. Any time He mentioned the cause of sickness or disease, He always attributed it to Satan.

No one really questions whether or not God CAN heal. (even atheists will admit that if there was a God, of course He would be able to heal or He wouldn't be much of a God.) Some Atheists are actually "one up" on some Christians in this respect. The doubt comes in when God's WILLINGNESS to heal is brought up. Any time the topic of God's willingness to heal came up, Jesus always said the same thing, "I will".

## Is Healing Always God's Will?

*Matt. 8:2-3* – *2. And, behold, there came a leper and worshipped him, saying, Lord, if thou wilt, thou canst make me clean. 3. And Jesus put forth his hand, and touched him, saying, I will; be thou clean. And immediately his leprosy was cleansed. (KJV)*

*Matt 8:2-3* – *2. A man with leprosy came and knelt before him and said, "Lord, if you are willing, you can make me clean." 3. Jesus reached out his hand and touched the man. "I am* willing," he said. "Be clean!" Immediately he was cured of his leprosy. (NIV)

**Matt 8:2-3** – 2. And behold, a leper came and worshiped Him, saying, "Lord, if You are willing, You can make me clean." 3. Jesus put out His hand and touched him, saying, "I am willing; be cleansed." Immediately his leprosy was cleansed. (NKJV)

**Matt 8:2-3** – And a leper came to Him and bowed down before Him, and said, "Lord, if You are willing, You can make me clean." Jesus stretched out His hand and touched him, saying, "I am willing; be cleansed." And immediately his leprosy was cleansed. (NASB)

**Matt 8:2-3** - Look! A leper is approaching. He kneels before him, worshiping. "Sir," the leper pleads, "if you want to, you can heal me." Jesus touches the man. "I want to," he says. "Be healed." And instantly the leprosy disappears. (TLB)

*"I Will"*

Strong's #2309 *thelo*, NT:2309

*Thelo* (thel'-o); or *ethelo* (eth-el'-o); in certain tenses *theleo* (thel-eh'-o); and *etheleo* (eth-el-eh'-o); which are otherwise obsolete; apparently strengthened from the alternate form of NT:138; to determine (as an active option from subjective impulse;

*"whereas"* NT:1014 properly denotes rather a passive acquiescence in objective considerations), i.e. choose or prefer (literally or figuratively); by implication, to wish, i.e. be inclined to (sometimes adverbially, gladly); impersonally for the future tense, to be about to; by Hebraism, to delight in: showing a disposition of the nature, and is in a continuous sense, and can be translated: "I am always willing". KJV-desire, be disposed (forward), intend, (be) will.

Strong's #2309-*thelo* or *ethelo* in certain tenses; *theleo* and *etheleo* which are otherwise obsolete – to will, to have in mind, to intend, to be resolved or determined, to purpose, to desire, to wish, to love, to like to do a thing, to be fond of doing, to take delight in, to have pleasure in.

(Note: To choose this word rather than #1014 shows the purposeful intent and determination rather than just saying, "whatever happens, happens".) Jesus was not just saying, "I

50

will do it." He was saying, "I will always do it because it is my intense desire and longing to act on my nature which is to deliver."

KJV-"*desire*", be disposed (forward), intend, list, love, mean, please, have rather, (be) will (have, -ling, -ling [-ly]).

## Does Anyone Ever Get Healed?

The above verses prove that people have been healed. I can provide many hundreds of instances of divine healing through faith in Jesus, both in my immediate family and in many other people's lives.

## Why or Why Not?

The reason anyone is not saved or healed is answered above, they would not do what it takes to find out what to do to be saved or healed, or if they did find out, they would not live by it. In either case it is still unbelief.

It is amazing to me that people today are still debating over God's will to heal any and all, when Jesus healed any and all and He was the full expression of God's will.

It seems that some believe that people were healed because they deserved it, and that people were better back then, so more people deserved it.

Or they think that Jesus just went around healing everyone because He was showing that He was God. If that were true He would not have told many of the people that He healed, not to say anything about how they were healed.

The truth is that Jesus healed everyone that would let Him heal them by their believing that He could and He will still do the same today.

# CHAPTER 5

## DIVINE HEALING BY FAITH

**Who Can Have "Great Faith"?**

**Jesus Only Commended Two People's Faith as Being "Great"- Neither Of Which Were In Covenant With God.**

*Matt. 8: 5-13 – And when Jesus was entered into Capernaum, there came unto him a centurion, beseeching him, 6. And saying, Lord, my servant lieth at home sick of the palsy, grievously tormented. 7. And Jesus saith unto him, I will come and heal him. 8. The centurion answered and said, Lord, I am not worthy that thou shouldest come under my roof: but speak the word only, and my servant shall be healed. 9. For I am a man under authority, having soldiers under me: and I say to this man, Go, and he goeth; and to another, Come, and he cometh; and to my servant, Do this, and he doeth it. 10. When Jesus heard it, he marvelled, and said to them that followed, Verily I say unto you, I have not found so great faith, no, not in Israel. 11. And I say unto you, That many shall come from the east and west, and shall sit down with Abraham, and Isaac, and*

Jacob, in the kingdom of heaven. 12. But the children of the kingdom shall be cast out into outer darkness: there shall be weeping and gnashing of teeth. 13. And Jesus said unto the centurion, Go thy way; and as thou hast believed, so be it done unto thee. And his servant was healed in the selfsame hour.

**Matt 15:22-28** – And, behold, a woman of Canaan came out of the same coasts, and cried unto him, saying, Have mercy on me, O Lord, thou Son of David; my daughter is grievously vexed with a devil. 23. But he answered her not a word. And his disciples came and besought him, saying, Send her away; for she crieth after us. 24. But he answered and said, I am not sent but unto the lost sheep of the house of Israel. 25. Then came she and worshipped him, saying, Lord, help me. 26. But he answered and said, It is not meet to take the children's bread, and to cast it to dogs. 27. And she said, Truth, Lord: yet the dogs eat of the crumbs which fall from their masters' table. 28. Then Jesus answered and said unto her, O woman, great is thy faith: be it unto thee even as thou wilt. And her daughter was made whole from that very hour.

**Luke 7:2-16** – And a certain centurion's servant, who was dear unto him, was sick, and ready to die. 3. And when he heard of Jesus, he sent unto him the elders of the Jews, beseeching him that he would come and heal his servant. 4. And when they came to Jesus, they besought him instantly, saying, That he was worthy for whom he should do this: 5. For he loveth our nation, and he hath built us a synagogue. 6. Then Jesus went with them. And when he was now not far from the house, the centurion sent friends to him, saying unto him, Lord, trouble not thyself: for I am not worthy that thou shouldest enter under my roof: 7. Wherefore neither thought I myself worthy to come unto thee: but say in a word, and my servant shall be healed. 8. For I also am a man set under authority, having under me soldiers, and I say unto one, Go, and he goeth; and to another, Come, and he cometh; and to my servant, Do this, and he doeth it. 9. When Jesus heard these things, he marvelled at him, and turned him about, and said unto the people that followed him, I say unto you, I have not found so great faith, no, not in Israel. 10. And they that were sent, returning to the house, found the servant whole that had been sick. 11. And it came to pass the day after, that he went into a city called Nain; and many of his disciples went with him, and much people. 12. Now when he came nigh to the gate of the city, behold, there was a dead man carried out, the only son of his mother, and she was a widow: and much people of the city was with her. 13. And when the Lord saw her, he had compassion on her, and said unto her, Weep not. 14. And he came and touched the bier: and they that bare him stood still. And he said, Young man, I say unto thee, Arise. 15. And he that was dead sat up, and began to speak. And he delivered him to his mother. 16. And there came a fear on all: and they glorified God, saying, That a great prophet is risen up among us; and, That God hath visited his people.

**Matt 9:20-22** – And, behold, a woman, which was diseased with an issue of blood twelve years, came behind him, and touched the hem of his garment: 21. For she said within herself, If I may but touch his garment, I shall be whole. 22. But Jesus turned him about, and when he saw her, he said, Daughter, be of good comfort; thy faith hath made thee whole. And the woman was made whole from that hour.

**Matt 9:27-30** – And when Jesus departed thence, two blind men followed him, crying, and saying, Thou Son of David, have mercy on us. 28. And when he was come into the house, the blind men came to him: and Jesus saith unto them, Believe ye that I am able to do this? They said unto him, Yea, Lord. 29. Then touched he their eyes, saying, According to your faith be it unto you. 30. And their eyes were opened; and Jesus straitly charged them, saying, See that no man know it.

*Matt 17:14-21 – And when they were come to the multitude, there came to him a certain man, kneeling down to him, and saying, 15. Lord, have mercy on my son: for he is lunatick, and sore vexed: for ofttimes he falleth into the fire, and oft into the water. 16. And I brought him to thy disciples, and they could not cure him. 17. Then Jesus answered and said, O faithless and perverse generation, how long shall I be with you? how long shall I suffer you? bring him hither to me. 18. And Jesus rebuked the devil; and he departed out of him: and the child was cured from that very hour. 19. Then came the disciples to Jesus apart, and said, Why could not we cast him out? 20. And Jesus said unto them, Because of your unbelief: for verily I say unto you, If ye have faith as a grain of mustard seed, ye shall say unto this mountain, Remove hence to yonder place; and it shall remove; and nothing shall be impossible unto you. 21. Howbeit this kind goeth not out but by prayer and fasting.*

*Matt 21:18-22 – Now in the morning as he returned into the city, he hungered. 19. And when he saw a fig tree in the way, he came to it, and found nothing thereon, but leaves only, and said unto it, Let no fruit grow on thee henceforward for ever. And presently the fig tree withered away. 20. And when the disciples saw it, they marvelled, saying, How soon is the fig tree withered away! 21. Jesus answered and said unto them, Verily I say unto you, If ye have faith, and doubt not, ye shall not only do this which is done to the fig tree, but also if ye shall say unto this mountain, Be thou removed, and be thou cast into the sea; it shall be done. 22. And all things, whatsoever ye shall ask in prayer, believing, ye shall receive.*

**Mark 11:22** - *And Jesus answering saith unto them, Have faith in God.* (It means what it says, Have faith in God.)

**FAITH FOR HEALING IS NOTHING MORE THAN SEEING PEOPLE AS GOD SEES THEM AND THEN TREATING THEM AS GOD WOULD TREAT THEM.**

Can God command us to do what He Himself would not do, in the same circumstances?

Of course not. That would make God worse than a hypocrite.

# CHAPTER 6

## THE ABC'S OF A DIVINE HEALING MINISTRY

### Principles That Guarantee Healing

The Law of Sowing and Reaping: Simply stated is this: What you plant is what will grow. Everything you say or do is planting. Make sure what you are planting is what you want to grow.

Remember, no seed returns one for one, if it did it would soon be extinct. Seeds always return multiplied. (30, 60, 100 fold) ("Fold" means: multiplied times over)

Scripture references:

*Gal. 6:7-10* – *Be not deceived; God is not mocked: for whatsoever a man soweth, that shall he also reap. 8. For he that soweth to his flesh shall of the flesh reap corruption; but he that soweth to the Spirit shall of the Spirit reap life everlasting. 9. And let us not be weary in well doing: for in due season we shall reap, if we faint not. 10. As we have therefore opportunity,* let us do good unto all men, especially unto them who are of the household of faith.

*Gen 8:22* – While the earth remaineth, seedtime and harvest, and cold and heat, and summer and winter, and day and night shall not cease.

*Matt 16:27* – For the Son of man shall come in the glory of his Father with his angels; and then he shall reward every man according to his works.

*Mark 9:41-42* – For whosoever shall give you a cup of water to drink in my name, because ye belong to Christ, verily I say unto you, he shall not lose his reward. 42. And whosoever shall offend one of these little ones that believe in me, it is better for him that a millstone were hanged about his neck, and he were cast into the sea. (KJV)

*Luke 6:31-38* - And as ye would that men should do to you, do ye also to them likewise. 32. For if ye love them which love you, what thank have ye? for sinners also love those that love them. 33. And if ye do good to them which do good to you, what thank have ye? for sinners also do even the same. 34. And if ye lend to them of whom ye hope to receive, what thank have ye? for sinners also lend to sinners, to receive as much again. 35. But love ye your enemies, and do good, and lend, hoping for nothing again; and your reward shall be great, and ye shall be the children of the Highest: for he is kind unto the unthankful and to the evil. 36. Be ye therefore merciful, as your Father also is merciful. 37. Judge not, and ye shall not be judged: condemn not, and ye shall not be condemned: forgive, and ye shall be forgiven: 38. Give, and it shall be given unto you; good measure, pressed down, and shaken together, and running over, shall men give into your bosom. For with the same measure that ye mete withal it shall be measured to you again.

**1 Cor. 3:7-10** – So then neither is he that planteth any thing, neither he that watereth; but God that giveth the increase. 8. Now he that planteth and he that watereth are one: and every man shall receive his own reward according to his own labour. 9. For we are labourers together with God: ye are God's husbandry, ye are God's building. 10. According to the grace of God which is given unto me, as a wise masterbuilder, I have laid the foundation, and another buildeth thereon. But let every man take heed how he buildeth thereupon.

***Col. 3:23-25** – And whatsoever ye do, do it heartily, as to the Lord, and not unto men; 24. Knowing that of the Lord ye shall receive the reward of the inheritance: for ye serve the Lord Christ. 25. But he that doeth wrong shall receive for the wrong which he hath done: and there is no respect of persons.*

***1 Tim 5:18** - For the scripture saith, Thou shalt not muzzle the ox that treadeth out the corn. And, The labourer is worthy of his reward.*

***2 Tim 4:14** – 14. Alexander the coppersmith did me much evil: the Lord reward him according to his works:*

***Heb 2:2-3** - 2For if the word spoken by angels was stedfast, and every transgression and disobedience received a just recompence of reward; 3. How shall we escape, if we neglect so great salvation; which at the first began to be spoken by the Lord, and was confirmed unto us by them that heard him;*

***Rev 22:12** – And, behold, I come quickly; and my reward is with me, to give every man according as his work shall be.*

**THE GOLDEN RULE.**

*Luke 6:31 – And as ye would that men should do to you, do ye also to them likewise*

The Law of the Spirit of Life in Christ Jesus:

Rom. 8:1-2 – 1. There is therefore now no condemnation to them which are in Christ Jesus, who walk not after the flesh, but after the Spirit. 2. For the law of the Spirit of life in Christ Jesus hath made me free from the law of sin and death.

**Three Steps to Action:**

Revelation- Enlightenment concerning God's Will (Oh, that's what God wants me to do, to be, etc.)

Conviction- determining where you are in fulfilling God's Will (Oh, I'm not anywhere near that.)

Action- completing the fulfillment of God's Will (I must do…)

## The ABC's of a Divine Healing Ministry

### A--Availability

*2 Chron 16:9* – *For the eyes of the LORD run to and fro throughout the whole earth, to shew himself strong in the behalf of them whose heart is perfect toward him. Herein thou hast done foolishly: therefore from henceforth thou shalt have wars.*

*Isa 6:8-9* – *Also I heard the voice of the Lord, saying, Whom shall I send, and who will go for us? Then said I, Here am I; send me. 9. And he said, Go, and tell this people, Hear ye indeed, but understand not; and see ye indeed, but perceive not.*

*Ezek 22:30* - *And I sought for a man among them, that should make up the hedge, and stand in the gap before me for the land, that I should not destroy it: but I found none.*

*Ezek 3:18-21* – *When I say unto the wicked, Thou shalt surely die; and thou gives him not warning, nor speaks to warn the wicked from his wicked way, to save his life; the same wicked man shall die in his iniquity; but his blood will I require at thine hand. 19. Yet if thou warn the wicked, and he turn not*

64

*from his wickedness, nor from his wicked way, he shall die in his iniquity; but thou hast delivered thy soul. 20. Again, When a righteous man doth turn from his righteousness, and commit iniquity, and I lay a stumbling block before him, he shall die: because thou hast not given him warning, he shall die in his sin, and his righteousness which he hath done shall not be remembered; but his blood will I require at thine hand. 21. Nevertheless if thou warn the righteous man, that the righteous sin not, and he doth not sin, he shall surely live, because he is warned; also thou hast delivered thy soul.*

***Ezek 33:3-9** – If when he seeth the sword come upon the land, he blow the trumpet, and warn the people; 4. Then whosoever heareth the sound of the trumpet, and taketh not warning; if the sword come, and take him away, his blood shall be upon his own head. 5. He heard the sound of the trumpet, and took not warning; his blood shall be upon him. But he that taketh warning shall deliver his soul. 6. But if the watchman see the sword come, and blow not the trumpet, and the people be not warned; if the sword come, and take any person from among them, he is taken away in his iniquity; but his blood will I require at the watchman's hand. 7. So thou, O son of man, I have set thee a watchman unto the house of Israel; therefore thou shalt hear the word at my mouth, and warn them from me.*

*8. When I say unto the wicked, O wicked man, thou shalt surely die; if thou dost not speak to warn the wicked from his way, that wicked man shall die in his iniquity; but his blood will I require at thine hand. 9. Nevertheless, if thou warn the wicked of his way to turn from it; if he do not turn from his way, he shall die in his iniquity; but thou hast delivered thy soul.*

**Prov 3:27-28** – *Withhold not good from them to whom it is due, when it is in the power of thine hand to do it. 28. Say not unto thy neighbour, Go, and come again, and to morrow I will give; when thou hast it.*

**James 4:17** – *Therefore to him that knoweth to do good and doeth it not, to him it is sin.*

Revelation- Enlightenment concerning God's Will - (Application- it is God's will for you to be available.)

Conviction- determining where you are in fulfilling God's Will - (Application- Are you available 24hours a day, 7days a week, ANYWHERE, or just on Sundays while you are at church where it is safe. Would you do in the grocery store what you do in Sunday service?)

Action- Completing the fulfillment of God's Will - (Application- Change, purposefully do something that you have not done before. Attack fear. Do what you know to do. Look for opportunity. Destroy fear and help man.

### B--Bold Believing

**Prov 28:1** – *The wicked flee when no man pursueth: but the righteous are bold as a lion.*

**1 Thess 2:2** –*But even after that we had suffered before, and were shamefully entreated, as ye know, at Philippi, we were bold in our God to speak unto you the gospel of God with much contention.*

**Eph 3:11-12** – *According to the eternal purpose which he purposed in Christ Jesus our Lord: 12. In whom we have boldness and access with confidence by the faith of him. (KJV)*

**1 John 4:17-18** – *Herein is our love made perfect, that we may have boldness in the day of judgment: because as he is, so are we in this world. 18. There is no fear in love; but perfect love casteth out fear: because fear hath torment. He that feareth is not made perfect in love.*

Revelation- Enlightenment concerning God's Will - (Application- it is God's Will that we be bold- meaning that we be outspoken concerning the gospel and the things of God.)

Conviction- Determining where you are in fulfilling God's Will - (Application- Are you as bold as God has made provision to be? Are you as willing to boldly believe that God will do what He said He would do?)

Action- completing the fulfillment of God's Will - (Application- Begin to find ways (situations) to be bold. Stretch to believe more boldly.

### C--Compassion

*Matt. 9:36-10:1* – *But when he saw the multitudes, he was moved with compassion on them, because they fainted, and were scattered abroad, as sheep having no shepherd. 37. Then saith he unto his disciples, The harvest truly is plenteous, but the labourers are few; 38. Pray ye therefore the Lord of the harvest, that he will send forth labourers into his harvest. Matthew 10:1 And when he had called unto him his twelve disciples, he gave them power against unclean spirits, to cast them out, and to heal all manner of sickness and all manner of disease.*

*__Matt 14:14__ – And Jesus went forth, and saw a great multitude, and was moved with compassion toward them, and he healed their sick.*

*__Matt 15:32__ – Then Jesus called his disciples unto him, and said, I have compassion on the multitude, because they continue with me now three days, and have nothing to eat: and I will not send them away fasting, lest they faint in the way.*

*__Matt 20:34__ – So Jesus had compassion on them, and touched their eyes: and immediately their eyes received sight, and they followed him.*

*__Mark 1:41__ –. And Jesus, moved with compassion, put forth his hand, and touched him, and saith unto him, I will; be thou clean.*

*__Mark 5:19__ – Howbeit Jesus suffered him not, but saith unto him, Go home to thy friends, and tell them how great things the Lord hath done for thee, and hath had compassion on thee.*

***Mark 6:34*** – *And Jesus, when he came out, saw much people, and was moved with compassion toward them, because they were as sheep not having a shepherd: and he began to teach them many things.*

***Mark 8:2-3*** – *I have compassion on the multitude, because they have now been with me three days, and have nothing to eat: 3. And if I send them away fasting to their own houses, they will faint by the way: for divers of them came from far.*

***Mark 9:22-27*** – *. And ofttimes it hath cast him into the fire, and into the waters, to destroy him: but if thou canst do any thing, have compassion on us, and help us. 23. Jesus said unto him, If thou canst believe, all things are possible to him that believeth. 24. And straightway the father of the child cried out, and said with tears, Lord, I believe; help thou mine unbelief. 25. When Jesus saw that the people came running together, he rebuked the foul spirit, saying unto him, Thou dumb and deaf spirit, I charge thee, come out of him, and enter no more into him. 26. And the spirit cried, and rent him sore, and came out of him: and he was as one dead; insomuch that many said, He is dead. 27. But Jesus took him by the hand, and lifted him up; and he arose.*

*Luke 7:13-15* – *And when the Lord saw her, he had compassion on her, and said unto her, Weep not. 14. And he came and touched the bier: and they that bare him stood still. And he said, Young man, I say unto thee, Arise. 15. And he that was dead sat up, and began to speak. And he delivered him to his mother.*

Revelation- Enlightenment concerning God's Will. - Application- God's will must be that I have compassion on people as my Lord did, and compassion always led (and leads) to the action to change their situation.

Conviction – Determining where you are in fulfilling God's Will. - Application – How often am I "overtaken" by compassion to help alleviate someone's problem?

Action – Completing the fulfillment of God's Will - Application – I must begin today to look at people through God's eyes and then begin to treat them as He would treat them. Compassion is the unction/desire to move. Moving is the expression of compassion. Today I will be moved by compassion and act.

# CHAPTER 7

## SONS OF GOD ACTING LIKE SONS OF GOD

### A Look At Spiritual Dominion

*Eph 4:11-15* –. *And he gave some, apostles; and some, prophets; and some, evangelists; and some, pastors and teachers; 12. For the perfecting of the saints, for the work of the ministry, for the edifying of the body of Christ: 13. Till we all come in the unity of the faith, and of the knowledge of the Son of God, unto a perfect man, unto the measure of the stature of the fulness of Christ: 14. That we henceforth be no more children, tossed to and fro, and carried about with every wind of doctrine, by the sleight of men, and cunning craftiness, whereby they lie in wait to deceive; 15. But speaking the truth in love, may grow up into him in all things, which is the head, even Christ: (KJV)*

### Who are Sons of God?

Adam:

*Luke 3:38* – *Which was the son of Enos, which was the son of Seth, which was the son of Adam, which was the son of God.*

Angels:

*Gen 6:2-4* – *That the sons of God saw the daughters of men that they were fair; and they took them wives of all which they chose. 3. And the LORD said, My spirit shall not always strive with man, for that he also is flesh: yet his days shall be an hundred and twenty years. 4. There were giants in the earth in those days; and also after that, when the sons of God came in unto the daughters of men, and they bare children to them, the same became mighty men which were of old, men of renown.*

*Job 1:6-7* – *Now there was a day when the sons of God came to present themselves before the LORD, and Satan came also among them. 7. And the LORD said unto Satan, Whence comest thou? Then Satan answered the LORD, and said, From going to and fro in the earth, and from walking up and down in it. KJV*

3. **Job 2:1** – 1. *Again there was a day when the sons of God came to present themselves before the LORD, and Satan came also among them to present himself before the LORD.*

4. **Job 38:7** – *When the morning stars sang together, and all the sons of God shouted for joy?*

Jesus:

**1 Jn 3:8** – *He that committeth sin is of the devil; for the devil sinneth from the beginning. For this purpose the Son of God was manifested, that he might destroy the works of the devil.*

Christians:

**1 John 3:1-3** – *Behold, what manner of love the Father hath bestowed upon us, that we should be called the sons of God: therefore the world knoweth us not, because it knew him not. 2. Beloved, now are we the sons of God, and it doth not yet appear what we shall be: but we know that, when he shall appear, we shall be like him; for we shall see him as he is. 3. And every man that hath this hope in him purifieth himself, even as he is pure.*

*Phil 2:15-16* – *That ye may be blameless and harmless, the sons of God, without rebuke, in the midst of a crooked and perverse nation, among whom ye shine as lights in the world; 16. Holding forth the word of life; that I may rejoice in the day of Christ, that I have not run in vain, neither laboured in vain.*

*Rom 8:18-21* – *For I reckon that the sufferings of this present time are not worthy to be compared with the glory which shall be revealed in us. 19. For the earnest expectation of the creature waiteth for the manifestation of the sons of God. 20. For the creature was made subject to vanity, not willingly, but by reason of him who hath subjected the same in hope, 21. Because the creature itself also shall be delivered from the bondage of corruption into the glorious liberty of the children of God.*

*John 1:12* – *But as many as received him, to them gave he power to become the sons of God, even to them that believe on his name:*

## What Position Do Sons of God Occupy?

A position of Dominion:

*Gen 1:26-28 – And God said, Let us make man in our image, after our likeness: and let them have dominion (#7287) over the fish of the sea, and over the fowl of the air, and over the cattle, and over all the earth, and over every creeping thing that creepeth upon the earth. 27. So God created man in his own image, in the image of God created he him; male and female created he them. 28. And God blessed them, and God said unto them, Be fruitful, and multiply, and replenish the earth, and subdue it: and have dominion (#7287) over the fish of the sea, and over the fowl of the air, and over every living thing that moveth upon the earth.*

What is "dominion"?

Strong's #7287 *radah* (raw-daw'); to tread down, i.e. subjugate; specifically, to crumble off: translated in the KJV as: (to make to) have dominion, to prevail against, reign, (bear, to make to) rule over, take.

Brown/Driver/Brigg's #7287 *radah*- 1)to rule, to have dominion, to dominate, to tread down –a) to have dominion, to rule, to subjugate –b) to cause to dominate.

*Ps 8:4-8* – *What is man, that thou art mindful of him? and the son of man, that thou visitest him? 5. For thou hast made him a little lower than the angels, and hast crowned him with glory and honour. 6. Thou madest him to have dominion (#4910) over the works of thy hands; thou hast put all things under his feet: 7. All sheep and oxen, yea, and the beasts of the field; 8. The fowl of the air, and the fish of the sea, and whatsoever passeth through the paths of the seas.*

Strong's #4910 *mashal* (maw-shal'); to rule: translated in the KJV as: (have, make to have) dominion, governor, reign, (to cause to have) rule, have power.

Brown/Driver/Brigg's #4910 *mashal* – to rule, to have dominion, to reign; to rule, to have dominion 1) to cause to rule, 2) to exercise dominion.

A position of Authority – As one with authority – over diseases, sicknesses, devils.

*Isa 45:11* – *Thus saith the LORD, the Holy One of Israel, and his Maker, Ask me of things to come concerning my sons, and concerning the work of my hands command ye me. (KJV)*

78

**Matt 7:28-29** (referring to Jesus) – *And it came to pass, when He had ended these sayings, the people were astonished at his doctrine: 29. For he taught them as one having authority, and not as the scribes.*

**Matt 28:18-20** (referring to both Jesus and Man) – *And He came and spoke unto them, saying, All power is given unto me in heaven and in earth. 19. Go ye therefore, and teach all nations, baptizing them in the name of the Father, and of the Son, and of the Holy Ghost: 20. Teaching them to observe all things whatsoever I have commanded you: and, lo, I am with you always, even unto the end of the world. Amen.*

**Mark 6:7** (referring to man) – *7. And he called unto him the twelve, and began to send them forth by two and two; and gave them power over unclean spirits;*

**Matt 9:37-10:1**(referring to man) – *37. Then saith he unto his disciples, The harvest truly is plenteous, but the labourers are few; 38. Pray ye therefore the Lord of the harvest, that he will send forth labourers into his harvest. 10:1 And when he had called unto him his twelve disciples, he gave them power against unclean spirits, to cast them out, and to heal all manner of sickness and all manner of disease. (KJV)*

A position of Responsibility / Duty – A position of servant to all but master to devils.

*Mark 10:44-45 – And whosoever of you will be the chiefest, shall be servant of all. 45. For even the Son of man came not to be ministered unto, but to minister, and to give his life a ransom for many.*

*Matt 7:12 –. Therefore all things whatsoever ye would that men should do to you, do ye even so to them: for this is the law and the prophets.*

*Luke 17:10 – So likewise ye, when ye shall have done all those things which are commanded you, say, We are unprofitable servants: we have done that which was our duty to do.*

*James 4:17 – Therefore to him that knoweth to do good, and doeth it not, to him it is sin.*

## What Does A Son of God Act Like?

The attributes of Jesus:

The Fruit of the Spirit:

*Gal 5:22-25 – But the fruit of the Spirit is love, joy, peace, longsuffering, gentleness, goodness, faith, 23. meekness, temperance: against such there is no law. 24. And they that are Christ's have crucified the flesh with the affections and lusts. 25. If we live in the Spirit, let us also walk in the Spirit.*

The Gifts of the Spirit:

*1 Cor 12:8-10 – For to one is given by the Spirit the word of wisdom; to another the word of knowledge by the same Spirit; 9. To another the gifts of healing by the same Spirit; 10. To another the working of miracles; to another prophecy; to another discerning of spirits' to another diverse kinds of tongues; to another the interpretation of tongues:*

Does what please the Father:

*John 8:29 – And he that sent me is with me: the Father hath not left me alone; for I do always those things that please him.*

Speaks the words of The Father:

*John 3:34* - *For he whom God hath sent speaketh the words of God giveth not the Spirit by measure unto him.*

Does the works of The Father:

See John 8:29 (above)

Destroys the works of the devil:

*1 John 3:8* – *He that committeth sin is of the devil; for the devil sinneth from the beginning. For this purpose the Son of God was manifested, that he might destroy the works of the devil.*

*Acts 10:38* – *How God anointed Jesus of Nazareth with the Holy Ghost and with power: who went about doing good, and healing all that were oppressed of the devil; for God was with him.*

*John 10:10* – *The thief cometh not, but for to steal, and to kill, and to destroy: I am come that they might have life, and that they might have it more abundantly.*

Seeks those that are lost:

*Luke 19:10* – *For the Son of man is come to seek and to save that which was lost.*

In the area of Spiritual Dominion, we need only see a few things clearly to change our lives AND the lives of all we meet forever. If you will earnestly seek to have the truths that I am about to share with you, engrafted into your heart, you will walk upon this earth like Jesus, as God intends you to.

**Truth #1** – God intended MAN to have and walk in dominion ON THE EARTH.

**Truth #2** – Man forfeited that position of dominion by acting on Satan's word instead of God's word.

**Truth #3** – When man forfeited his position of dominion, he also forfeited his position of fellowship and communion. (Fellowship, Communion, and Dominion are not different positions, they are all one in the same.)

**Truth #4** – God wanted man in a position of fellowship/dominion so much that He was willing to sacrifice Jesus to return man to his original position.

**Truth #5** – Jesus came to destroy the works of the devil – By His life He showed us how to live on earth as a man walking in dominion. He was the second Adam. Jesus walked like a man without sin, in a sinful world.

**Truth #6** – Jesus did His part. If we are not back into our original position before God, then Jesus' sacrifice was not as good as Adam's sin was bad.

**Truth #7** – We, being the body of Christ, are to walk as Jesus upon the earth, being for others what Jesus was and is for us. We are to be deliverers of those who are bound by Satan, as Jesus did. Jesus showed us how. By having fellowship and communion with our Heavenly Father, and freely giving what we have freely received.

**Examples of Dominion given to man:**

Freedom to heal anyone.

*Matt 10:7-8* - *And as ye go, preach, saying, The kingdom of heaven is at hand. 8. Heal the sick, cleanse the lepers, raise the dead, cast out devils: freely ye have received, freely give.*

*Luke 9:1-2* – Then he called his twelve disciples together, and gave them power and authority over all devils, and to cure diseases. 2. And he sent them to preach the kingdom of God, and to heal the sick.

*Luke 9:4-6* – And whatsoever house ye enter into, there abide, and thence depart. 5. And whosoever will not receive you, when ye go out of that city, shake off the very dust from your feet for a testimony against them. 6. And they departed, and went through the towns, preaching the gospel, and healing everywhere.

*Luke 10:8-9* – And into whatsoever city ye enter, and they receive you, eat such things as are set before you: 9. And heal the sick that are therein, and say unto them, The kingdom of God is come nigh unto you.

Freedom to pray for anything within the parameters of a Christian life.

*Matt 16:19* – And I will give unto thee the keys of the kingdom of heaven: and whatsoever thou shalt bind on earth shall be bound in heaven: and whatsoever thou shalt loose on earth shall be loosed in heaven.

*Matt 21:21-22* – *Jesus answered and said unto them, Verily I say unto you, If ye have faith, and doubt not, ye shall not only do this which is done to the fig tree, but also if ye shall say unto this mountain, Be thou removed, and be thou cast into the sea; it shall be done. 22. And all things, whatsoever ye shall ask in prayer, believing, ye shall receive.*

Freedom to say what you want and get it.

*Mark 11:23-24* – *For verily I say unto you, That whosoever shall say unto this mountain, Be thou removed, and be thou cast into the sea; and shall not doubt in his heart, but shall believe that those things which he saith shall come to pass; he shall have whatsoever he saith. 24. Therefore I say unto you, What things soever ye desire, when ye pray, believe that ye receive them, and ye shall have them.*

# CHAPTER 8:

---

## THE SECRET KEY TO A DIVINE HEALING MINISTRY

**The most frustrating position in which Christians that believe in divine healing can find themselves, is to know that God can heal, that God does heal and that He will heal the sick, and to know the "A, B, C's" of divine healing ministry: availability, boldness, and compassion, and yet still not be used of God to heal the sick.**

Christians everywhere are looking for that one book that can give them what they need to get started in healing ministry.

They are looking for that one key that will instantly change everything.

They think (and are often taught) that if they hear enough "Word" preaching, they will gradually get filled up with faith and then they will explode upon the world scene as the next world-renowned healing evangelist.

They think that if they just get that new book out by the man with that great healing ministry, they will "get it".

That is their problem. They are trying to get "it" rather than get "Him"

**The # 1 secret of a healing ministry:**

*Acts 4:13* - *Now when they saw the boldness of Peter and John, and perceived that they were unlearned and ignorant men, they marveled: and they took knowledge of them that they had been with Jesus.*

The first secret key is to know that there is no secret key.

Availability is an important key, but without it you could still be used by God to heal the sick. Boldness is an important key, but without it you could still be used by God to heal the sick. Compassion is an important key, but without it you could still be used by God to heal the sick, at least for a while.

But without having been with Jesus, your ministry to heal the sick will be weak, unproductive, and short lived.

Availability can be produced deciding to be available.

Boldness can be a natural tendency you already possess, or it can come through being convinced that you must do a particular thing.

Compassion can be the "natural" outflow of the nature of God in a Christian life.

Many Christians are compassionate towards the sick, and try to alleviate their suffering using the natural remedies of medical science. But when a Christian begins to spend time with God, they begin to think, and act like Him.

The answer is not usually in major changes, most often it is minor adjustments that makes a major difference.

Many times when things are not going the way we believe they should, we begin to make major changes. While we are making the big changes, we often overlook the few small things that would have made a big difference if we had just made the adjustments.

If you are a Christian, you are probably trying to serve God. It is unlikely that you should, could, or would make large sweeping changes even if they were needed. It is like taking medicine or vitamins, if you begin taking several different kinds at the same time, you will have no way of knowing what each individual ingredient did. It would be better to start taking them one at a time so that you can tell what effect each one had on your body.

If you are **available, bold and compassionate,** yet for some reason you are still not seeing the kind of flow of the Spirit of God in your life that you want to see, there are only a few things that could be standing in the way.

Hindrances to the Power of God in and through YOUR LIFE.

The first major hindrance to the power of God in a person's life is SIN. This shouldn't even have to be addressed. If you are a Christian you are steadily "mortifying" the deeds of the flesh. If you are a Christian, you have crucified that flesh and the lust thereof.

**Rom 8:13** - *For if ye live after the flesh, ye shall die: but if ye through the Spirit do mortify the deeds of the body, ye shall live.*

**Gal 5:24** - *And they that are Christ's have crucified the flesh with the affections and lusts.*

**I John 2:1** - *My little children, these things write I unto you, that ye sin not. And if any man sin, we have an advocate with the Father, Jesus Christ the righteous:*

The second major hindrance to the power of God is unbelief.

Unbelief can also be classified as sin, but we will look at it separately at this time.

Unbelief is nothing more than calling God a liar. Most people see unbelief as not knowing.

Unbelief is not "not knowing", it is "knowing" but choosing not to believe.

*Matt 13:57-58* – *And they were offended in him. But Jesus said unto them, A prophet is not without honour, save in his own country, and in his own house. 58. And he did not many mighty works there because of their unbelief.*

*Mark 6:3-6* – *Is not this the carpenter, the son of Mary, the brother of James, and Joses, and of Juda, and Simon? and are not his sisters here with us? And they were offended at him. 4. But Jesus said unto them, A prophet is not without honour, but in his own country, and among his own kin, and in his own house. 5. And he could there do no mighty work, save that he laid his hands upon a few sick folk, and healed them. 6. And he marvelled because of their unbelief. And he went round about the villages, teaching.*

Strong's #570 *apaistia* (ap-is-tee'-ah); From 571; faithlessness, i.e. (negatively) disbelief (lack of Christian faith), of (positively) unfaithfulness (disobedience): KJV – unbelief.

If you have had teaching concerning the will of God in the area of healing, and you know that it is always God's will to heal in answer to faith.

If you are not living in sin.

If you are not in unbelief, but are rather in belief, trusting God to honor His Word.

If you are Available to God to be used.

If you are Bold to speak up concerning God's desire to heal.

If you are Compassionate, walking in the love of God for people.

If all these things apply to you, and yet you still do not see God's power in your life, there can be ONLY one reason.

You are not spending enough time in prayer.

Missionary statesman John G. Lake believed that prayer was to the power of God what a dynamo is to electricity. He said that (strong, believing) prayer stirred up the power of God in a Christian's souls until there was nothing they could except but to be used of God.

In World War 2 America dropped an atomic bomb on two Japanese cities, Hiroshima and Nagasaki. After Japan surrendered, American medical personnel went in to help the Japanese ease the suffering of the survivors of the cities. Part of their process included taking measurements of the radioactivity of the survivors of the cities. The level of radioactivity each person had, helped them determine how close to "Ground – zero" they were. They could not determine how close they were by the severity of their radiation burns because burns could be less or worse depending upon what was between them and the blast. But radioactivity would remain the same regardless of what was between them, except for one substance, lead. Lead was the only effective shield against radiation.

Prayer (spending time in God's presence) is like being in one of those Japanese towns. The power of God in your life is a good indicator of how close to the Throne of God you have been and how long you were there.

The closer you get and the longer you stay there the more saturated you become.

The longer you stay in the presence of God, the more of his Spirit will remain with you in your daily life.

The longer you are out in the cold winter weather, the longer it will take for you to warm back up.

The more you stay in the atmosphere of this world, the longer it will take you to "warm up" to God. This is why we worship and pray to start church services. Since many people seem to live most of their time in the natural / flesh, etc., it sometimes takes a long time to enter the presence of God. Some people attend church and never get into the presence of God, because the only time they pray is in church.

*1 Thess 5:15-22 – See that none render evil for evil unto any man; but ever follow that which is good, both among yourselves, and to all men. 16. Rejoice evermore. 17. Pray without ceasing. 18. In every thing give thanks: for this is the will of God in Christ Jesus concerning you. 19. Quench not the Spirit. 20. Despise not prophesyings. 21. Prove all things; hold fast that which is good. 22. Abstain from all appearance of evil.*

When you read this scripture or bring up prayer, people automatically begin making excuses as to why they cannot do this. The first rule of Christianity is this. **We can do whatever God commands us to do,** or He would be unjust to require it of us. So first we must decide that we can pray without ceasing. Then we must decide that we will begin to pray without ceasing, if God will show us how. Next we must ask God for wisdom in how to pray without ceasing. When you ask, here is the answer that He will give you. Relationship. If you had a best friend that was always easy to get along with, always knew the answer to every question you asked, was always the ultimate joy to be around, how hard would it be to spend all your time talking AND listening to him? Well God is that friend. Once you begin to experience fellowship with God, you will find it very easy to spend all your time in His presence.

To fulfill the command to "pray without ceasing", we must first redefined the word "pray". If you think praying means always talking or always asking God for something, then yes you would have a hard time fulfilling this scripture. There are times when you should formally approach God with your petitions and requests, but most of the time you should just live in the presence of God. Many times I do not say Amen when I am talking to God during the day, because I don't want to leave His presence, so I just talk with Him and live with Him. He talks to me consistently, sharing insights into the Scriptures. Every sermon I preach and every lesson I teach is conceived in this manner. As you begin to live in this manner, you will notice your spiritual life literally explode with new revelation into the nature and character of God. What may look very hard, boring, and time-consuming, will become the most exciting time of your spiritual growth. Once you begin this lifestyle, you will be amazed at how fast you grow spiritually. I have had many people comment upon my spiritual understanding or wisdom. I know that I have not yet even scratched the surface of the spiritual depths that are in Christ Jesus. But everyday I learn more.

## How can you pray without ceasing?

Make sure everything you say could be used in prayer.

Begin to carry on a conversation with God.

Verbally ask God to reveal things to you. Ask God to answer your questions, to bring into manifestation the wisdom of Christ that has been placed in your spirit.

Begin to ask God to reveal things to you in the Bible.

Ask God to manifest the gifts of the Spirit in your life so that you can help others. The fastest way to receive from God is to share with others what God shares with you. (Make sure you give Him the credit for sharing it with you.)

Live in the presence of God. When you wake up in the morning say Good Morning Father, Son and Holy Ghost. When you lay down to go to sleep at night, say, Good Night, Father, Son and Holy Ghost.

Before you go to sleep, always ask God to talk to you in your sleep, and tell you the things that He couldn't get across to you while you were awake. When I began to do this, instantly God began doing mighty things in my sleep. My dreams are spiritual, I receive revelations and I never have nightmares or bad night's sleep (or a bad next day for that matter). My life is daily becoming more and more full of God.

**Pray in tongues. Pray loud, strong and hard.**

Remember, you are not ready for the battleground until you have been on the Holy Ground.

Pray everywhere, all the time. You cannot pray too much. Prayer is like scaring the crows away from your cornfield. It will keep Satan's doubts and temptation away. Then when you see someone needing a touch from God, you will be in the right "frame of mind" to give them that touch, because greater is He that is in you than he that is in the world. Remember, some people will never get any closer to God than when they have crossed your path.

# Part 2--The Seven Questions of Divine Healing

Chapter 1: Does God Heal?

Chapter 2: Who Does God Heal?

Chapter 3: When Does God Heal?

Chapter 4: Why Does God Heal?

Chapter 5: Where Does God Heal?

Chapter 6: How Does God Heal?

Chapter 7: What Does This Mean To You?

# Chapter 1:

## Does God Heal?

### Does God ever Heal?

God Has Healed in the Past.

***Genesis 20:17*** - *So Abraham prayed unto God: and God healed Abimelech, and his wife, and his maidservants; and they bare children.*

***Leviticus 13:18*** - *The flesh also, in which, even in the skin thereof, was a boil, and is healed,*

***Leviticus 13:37*** - *But if the scall be in his sight at a stay, and that there is black hair grown up therein; the scall is healed, he is clean: and the priest shall pronounce him clean.*

***1 Samuel 6:3*** - *And they said, If ye send away the ark of the God of Israel, send it not empty; but in any wise return him a trespass offering: then ye shall be healed, and it shall be known to you why his hand is not removed from you.*

*II Kings 2:21* - *And he went forth unto the spring of the waters, and cast the salt in there, and said, Thus saith the LORD, I have healed these waters; there shall not be from thence any more death or barren land.*

*2 Chronicles 30:20* - *And the LORD hearkened to Hezekiah, and healed the people.*

*Psalm 30:2* - *0 LORD my God, I cried unto thee, and thou hast healed me.*

*Psalm 107:20* - *He sent his word, and healed them, and delivered them from their destructions.*

*Isaiah 6:10* - *Make the heart of this people fat, and make their ears heavy, and shut their eyes; lest they see with their eyes, and hear with their ears, and understand with their heart, and convert, and be healed.*

*Isaiah 53:5* - *But he was wounded for our transgressions, he was bruised for our iniquities: the chastisement of our peace was upon him; and with his stripes we are healed.*

**Psalm 103:3** - *Who forgiveth all thine iniquities; who healeth all thy diseases;*

God has promised to Heal in the Future.

**Revelation 22:2** - *In the midst of the street of it, and on either side of the river, was there the tree of life, which bare twelve manner of fruits, and yielded her fruit every month: and the leaves of the tree were for the healing of the nations.*

God Never Changes.

**Malachi 3:6** - *For I am the LORD, I change not;*

**Hebrews 13:8** - *Jesus Christ the same yesterday, and to day, and for ever.*

**Common Fallacies**:

**Fallacy #1** - God Does Not Heal Today.

If God never changes - if He ever healed, He will heal again under the right circumstances. God cannot arbitrarily choose to heal one person and leave another sick, that would violate God's Word which tells us that He is not a respecter of persons.

He is a respecter of faith however, and to be totally fair He must make faith available to anyone.

Faith is the only requirement that God can require and remain just.

Faith is available to anyone that will "only believe".

**Romans 2:11** - *For there is no respect of persons with God.*

**Ephesians 6:9** - *And, ye masters, do the same things unto them, forbearing threatening: knowing that your Master also is in heaven; neither is there respect of persons with him.*

**Colossians 3:25** - *But he that doeth wrong shall receive for the wrong which he hath done: and there is no respect of persons.*

**Fallacy #2** - God Does Not Heal In This Current "Dispensation".

What dispensation is that? (See point 1 below - paragraph 4)

What dispensation are we in? (Again see point 1 below - paragraph 4)

Who categorized the dispensations? (Where, in the Bible, are the dispensations listed?) I am not disputing the reality of dispensations, just man's arrogance for deciding for God what He cannot or will not do.

In which of the "dispensations" has God stated that He would not heal?

The Apostle Peter categorized his day as "the last days" when he depicted the outpouring of the Holy Spirit on the Day of Pentecost as the beginning of the fulfillment of the prophecy spoken by the Prophet Joel (2:28).

*Acts 2:14-43 – But Peter, standing up with the eleven, lifted up his voice, and said unto them, Ye men of Judaea, and all ye that dwell at Jerusalem, be this known unto you, and hearken to my words: 15. For these are not drunken, as ye suppose, seeing it is but the third hour of the day. 16. But this is that which was spoken by the prophet Joel; 17. And it shall come to pass in the last days, saith God, I will pour out of my Spirit upon all flesh: and your sons and your daughters shall prophesy, and your young men shall see visions, and your old men shall dream dreams: 18. And on my servants and on my handmaidens I will pour out in those days of my Spirit; and they shall prophesy: 19. And I will shew wonders in heaven above, and signs in the earth beneath; blood, and fire, and vapor of smoke: 20. The sun shall be turned into darkness, and the moon into blood, before that great and notable day of the Lord come:*

*38. And it shall come to pass that whosoever shall call on the name of the Lord shall be saved.* (Are "men" still calling upon the Name of the Lord and being saved? If so, we must still be in "those days") *22. Ye men of Israel, hear these words; Jesus of Nazareth, a man approved of God among you by miracles and wonders and signs, which God did by him in the midst of you, as ye yourselves also know:* (This is still how God approves a man's ministry.) *32. This Jesus hath God raised up, whereof we all are witnesses. 33. Therefore being by the right hand of God exalted, and having received of the Father the promise of the Holy Ghost, he bath shed forth this, which ye*

108

*now see and hear. 37. Now when they heard this, they were pricked in their heart, and said unto Peter and to the rest of the apostles, Men and brethren, what shall we do? 38 Then Peter said unto them, Repent, and be baptized every one of you in the name of Jesus Christ for the remission of sins, and ye shall receive the gift of the Holy Ghost.* (Apparently, this is referring to what has just been witnessed by these men.) *39. For the promise* (the gift of the Holy Ghost) *is unto you, and to your children, and to all that are afar off even as many as the Lord our God shall call.* (As long as the Lord shall call people, they can receive the promise, the gift of the Holy Ghost.) *40. And with many other words did he testify and exhort, saying, Save yourselves from this untoward generation. 41. Then they that gladly received his word were baptized: and the same day there were added unto them about three thousand souls. 42. And they continued stedfastly in the apostles' doctrine and fellowship, and in breaking of bread, and in prayers.* (The above constituted the bulk of the Apostle's doctrine until, and following, the first Jerusalem council.) *43. And fear came upon every soul:* (This doesn't happen much anymore) *and many wonders and signs were done by the apostles.* (Probably because this doesn't happen much anymore.)

When did healing stop? - Church History

Healing and miracles have been recorded throughout Church history. As a matter of fact, there has never been a time when, somewhere in the earth, healings were not known to the church. If you begin to study church history you will find that those who were known to be fervent in faith toward God, were also known to experience miraculous healing and other gifts of the Spirit. When people began to turn their hearts toward God, He always responds by manifesting Himself through the same means He has always manifested Himself which is through signs and wonders.

If you begin to compare the dates of recorded miracles and healings you will also find that they will correspond with dates of revivals in the church. Even the leading figures of the well known Awakenings and Revivals were accustomed to the miraculous.

John Wesley recorded over 200 healings in his journals alone. Charles Finney recorded several healings and "miracles".

If one person, at any time, since the "Apostolic Days" has been healed, it proves God still heals.

God Heals Some But Doesn't Heal Others.

God is no respecter of persons - what He does for one He will do for another. (See Point 2.a)

This belief stems from a wrong conception of how and why God heals. (See later chap.)

☐

# Chapter 2:

## Who Does God Heal?

### Who Has God Healed?

Scriptural accounts of various types of people healed by God.

God has healed every type of person, from Kings to prostitutes, pagans to prophets.

### Who has God Promised to Heal?

Scriptural Healing Promises.

God has promised to heal anyone with faith.

*Luke 17:5-6* - *And the apostles said unto the Lord, Increase our faith. And the Lord said, If ye had faith as a grain of mustard seed, ye might say unto this sycamine tree, Be thou plucked up by the root, and be thou planted in the sea; and it should obey you.*

*Mark 11:22-24* - *And Jesus answering saith unto them, Have faith in God. 23. For verily I say unto you, That whosoever shall say unto this i4iouilain, Be thou removed, and be thou cast into the sea; and shall not doubt in his heart, but shall believe that those things which he saith shall come to pass; he shall have whatsoever he saith. 24. Therefore I say unto you, What things soever ye desire, when ye pray, believe that ye receive them, and ye shall have them.*

*Isaiah 57:17-19* - *For the iniquity of his covetousness was I wroth, and smote him: I hid me, and was wroth, and he went on frowardly in the way of his heart. 18. I have seen his ways, and will heal him: I will lead him also, and restore comforts unto him and to his mourners. 19. I create the fruit of the lips; Peace, peace to him that is far off, and to him that is near, saith the LORD; and I will heal him.*

*Matt 8:5-7* - *And when Jesus was entered into Capernaum, there came unto him a centurion, beseeching him, 6. And saying, Lord, my servant lieth at home sick of the palsy, grievously tormented. 7. And Jesus saith unto him, I will come and heal him.*

114

*Matt 13:15* - *For this people's heart is waxed gross, and their ears are dull of hearing, and their eyes they have closed; lest at any time they should see with their eyes, and hear with their ears, and should understand with their heart, and should be converted, and I should heal them.*

You can see by the above verses that God has promised to heal anyone that turns from their evil ways. By the following verses you can clearly see that in each instance it was their faith that caused their healing, not just the arbitrary "Will of God". In each example there was no other requirement or ingredient besides faith. Even those who were sick because of sin were healed and their sins forgiven. Jesus simply went around doing good and healing ALL that were oppressed of the devil. (Acts 10:38) He went about wiping the slate clean for each person that came for help.

*Matt 9:2* - *And, behold, they brought to him a man sick of the palsy, lying on a bed: and Jesus seeing their faith said unto the sick of the palsy; Son, be of good cheer; thy sins be forgiven thee.*

*Matt 9:22* - But Jesus turned him about, and when he saw her, he said. Daughter, be of good comfort: thy faith hath made thee whole. And the woman was made whole from that hour.

*Matt 9:29* - Then touched he their eyes, saying, According to your faith be it unto you.

*Matt 15:28* - Then Jesus answered and said unto her, O woman, great is thy faith: be it unto thee even as thou wilt. And her daughter was made whole from that very hour.

*Mark 2:5* - When Jesus saw their faith, he said unto the sick of the palsy, Son, thy sins be forgiven thee.

*Mark 5:34* - And he said unto her, Daughter, thy faith hath made thee whole; go in peace, and be whole of thy plague.

*Mark 10:52* - And Jesus said unto him, go thy way; thy faith hath made thee whole. And immediately he received his sight, and followed Jesus in the way.

*Luke 5:18-20* –. And, behold, men brought in a bed a man which was taken with a palsy: and they sought means to bring him in, and to lay him before him. 19. And when they could not find by what way they might bring him in because of the multitude, they went upon the housetop, and let him down through the tiling with his couch into the midst before Jesus. 20. And when he saw their faith, he said unto him, Man, thy sins are forgiven thee.

**Luke 7:50** - And he said to the woman, Thy Faith hath saved thee; go in peace.

**Luke 8:48** - And he said unto her, Daughter, be of good comfort: thy faith hath made thee whole; go in peace.

**Luke 17:19** - And he said unto him, Arise, go thy way: thy faith hath made thee whole.

**Luke 18:42** - And Jesus said unto him, Receive thy sight: thy faith hath saved thee.

**Acts 3:1-16** – Now Peter and John went up together into the temple at the hour of prayer, being the ninth hour. 2. And a certain man lame from his mother's womb was carried, whom they laid daily at the gate of the temple which is called Beautiful, to ask alms of them that entered into the temple; 3. Who seeing Peter and John about to go into the temple asked an alms. 4. And Peter, fastening his eyes upon him with John, said, Look on us. 5. And he gave heed unto them, expecting to receive something of them. 6. Then Peter said, Silver and gold have I none; but such as I have give I thee: In the name of Jesus Christ of Nazareth rise up and walk. 7. And he took him by the right hand, and lifted him up: and immediately his feet and ankle bones received strength. 8. And he leaping up stood, and walked, and entered with them into the temple, walking, and leaping, and praising God. 9. And all the people saw him walking and praising God: 10. And they knew that it was he which sat for alms at the Beautiful gate of the temple: and they were filled with wonder and amazement at that which had happened unto him. 11. And as the lame man which was healed held Peter and John, all the people ran together unto them in the porch that is called Solomon's, greatly wondering. 12. And when Peter saw it, he answered unto the people, Ye men of Israel, why marvel ye at this? or why look ye so earnestly on us, as though by our own power or holiness we had made this man to walk? 13. The God of Abraham, and of Isaac, and of Jacob, the God of our fathers, hath glorified his Son Jesus; whom ye delivered up, and denied him in the presence of Pilate, when he was determined to let him go. 14. But ye denied the Holy One and the Just, and desired a murderer to be granted unto you; 15. And killed the Prince of *life, whom God hath raised from the dead; whereof we are witnesses. 16. And his name through faith in his name hath made this man strong, whom ye see and know: yea, the faith which is by him lath given him this perfect soundness in the presence of you all.*

**"Whosoever" Means YOUsoever.**

We sing "Just as I am" - believing that God will accept us into His family "just as we are", yet we cannot believe He would heal us just as we are. We know we cannot be good enough to warrant being saved, but we somehow believe we can be good enough to warrant being healed.

We are very quick to put ourselves into the category of the "whosoever" concerning forgiveness of sins, salvation, and "going to Heaven", but when it comes to the "whosoever" for answered prayer and having the power of the Spirit of God demonstrated in our life, we, suddenly start backpedaling and trying to put all the responsibility on God.□

# Chapter 3:

## When Does God Heal?

### When Does God Promise To Heal?

When You Pray

*Mark 11:24* - *Therefore I say unto you, What things soever ye desire, when ye pray, believe that ye receive them, and ye shall have them.*

When You Believe

*Mark 11:22-24* - *And Jesus answering saith unto them, Have faith in God. 23. For verily I say unto you, That whosoever shall say unto this mountain, Be thou removed, and be thou cast into the sea; and shall not doubt in his heart, but shall believe that those things which he saith shall come to pass; he shall have whatsoever he saith. 24. Therefore I say unto you, What things soever ye desire, when ye pray, believe that ye receive them, and ye shall have them.*

C. When You Pray for Others

*James 5:16* - *Confess your faults one to another, and pray one for another, that ye may be healed. The effectual fervent prayer of a righteous man availeth much.*

When YOU call for the Elders and they pray the prayer of faith.

*James 5:14-15* – *Is any sick among you? let him call for the elders of the church; and let them pray over him, anointing him with oil in the name of the Lord: 15. And the prayer of faith shall save the sick, and the Lord shall raise him up; and if he have committed sins, they shall be forgiven him.* (KJV)

Notice: The Elders must pray the PRAYER of FAITH NOT the prayer of Doubt and UNBELIEF. This verse also says that if you have committed sins they will be forgiven. Unforgiven sin will not hinder your healing. But once you are healed you should *"go and sin no more lest a worse thing come upon you"*.

## When Did Healing Become a Fact?

At the Atonement.

*Malt 8:17* - *That it might be fulfilled which was spoken by Esaias the prophet, saying, Himself took our infirmities, and bare our sicknesses.*

This verse was applied to Jesus, yet it refers to events (healings) before the atonement.

*Isaiah 53:4-6* – *Surely he hath borne our grief 's, and carried our sorrows: yet we did esteem him stricken, smitten of God, and afflicted. 5 But he was wounded for our transgressions; he was bruised for our iniquities: the chastisement of our peace was upon him; and with his stripes we are healed. 6. All we like sheep have gone astray; we have turned every one to his own way; and the LORD hath laid on him the iniquity of us all.*

## Brazen Serpent - Jesus Lifted up.

First let's prove that Jesus linked Himself to the brass serpent that Moses lifted up in the wilderness.

*John 3:14-15* – *And as Moses lifted up the serpent in the wilderness, even so must the Son of man be lifted up: 15. That whosoever believeth in him should not perish, but have eternal life.*

Here we see Jesus using the brazen serpent as an example and a "shadow" or "type" of how He would be "lifted up". Now let's see what effect raising the brazen serpent in the wilderness had on the people of God. We should also point out that the reason the people were attacked by serpents was because they had sinned. Their sin was complaining. Could this be why so many people in the church today are sick? Have they complained and have not repented?

**Numbers 21:4-9** – *And they journeyed from mount Hor by the way of the Red sea, to compass the land of Edom: and the soul of the people was much discouraged because of the way.*

(Notice they became discouraged because of their hard journey. Most people today would say they had a reason to complain, they were discouraged, and things were not going well. But God still counted it as sin.)

*5.And the people spake against God, and against Moses. Wherefore have ye brought us up out of Egypt to die in the wilderness? for there is no bread, neither is there any water; and our soul loatheth this light bread.*

(The sin that caused so many to die was that they "spake against" God and His appointed leader.)

*6And the LORD sent fiery serpents among the people, and they bit the people; and much people of Israel died. 7. Therefore the people came to Moses, and said, We have sinned, for we have spoken against the LORD, and against thee; pray unto the LORD, that he take away the serpents from us. And Moses prayed for the people. 8. And the LORD said unto Moses, Make thee a fiery serpent, and set it upon a pole: and it shall come to pass, that every one that is bitten, when he looketh upon it, shall live. 9. And Moses made a serpent of brass, and put it upon a pole, and it came to pass, that if a serpent had bitten any man, when he beheld the serpent of brass, he lived.*

(The scripture says that God "sent" the fiery serpents. I have heard many people try to explain away this verse, trying to protect God's image. Some say "sent" in the Hebrew, is in the permissive tense which would mean that God allowed the fiery serpents to attack them. I have no real problem with that.

That would also imply that the sowing of sin would also cause a reaping of the consequences, which is a Biblical principle. But the fact is that even if God did literally send the fiery serpents (the consequences of sin) He would still be just because the people did sin. The Righteous Judge has a right to judge righteously. This would also show us how willing God is to forgive and heal once the sinner repents.)

**IV. The wine and the bread - if physical healing wasn't in the atonement we would not need the bread which represents His body.**

# Chapter 4:

## Why Does God Heal?

**God Heals Because It is His Nature to Save/Heal.**

It is God's nature to give good things not evil things. —

*James 1:17* - *Every good gift and every perfect gift is from above, and cometh down from the Father of lights, with whom is no variableness, neither shadow of turning.* (KJV)

*Matt 7:8-11* – *For everyone that asketh receiveth; and he that seeketh findeth; and to him that knocketh it shall be opened. 9. Or what man is there of you, whom if his son ask bread, will he give him a stone? 10. Or if he ask a fish, will he give him a serpent? 11. If ye then, being evil, know how to give good gifts unto your children, how much more shall your Father which is in heaven give good things to them that ask him?*

To give life abundantly

*John 10:10* - *The thief cometh not, but for to steal, and to kill, and to destroy: I am come that they might have life, and that they might have it more abundantly.*

Jesus referred to the people as "sick" and He as the "Physician"

*Matt 9:12* - *But when Jesus heard that, he said unto them, They that be whole need not a physician, but they that are sick.* (See also Luke 5:31)

Jesus classified the sick and the sinner under one category just as He identified the two categories in John 10:10 - *Mark 2:17* - *When Jesus heard it, he saith unto them, They that are whole have no need of the physician, but they that are sick: I came not to call the righteous, but sinners to repentance.*

Here Jesus specifically refers to Himself as the Physician - *Luke 4:23* - *And he said unto them, Ye will surely say unto me this proverb, Physician, heal thyself: whatsoever we have heard done in Capernaum, do also here in thy country.*

God's thoughts of you are only good

*Jeremiah 29:11-13* – *For I know the thoughts that I think toward you, saith the LORD, thoughts of peace, and not of evil, to give you an expected end. 12. Then shall ye call upon me, and ye shall go and pray unto me, and I will hearken unto you. 13. And ye shall seek me, and find me, when ye shall search for me with all your heart.*

God's Name is *Jehovah-Rapha* - Which means: "I AM the Lord that heals" - *Exod 15:26* - *And said, If thou wilt diligently hearken to the voice of the LORD thy God, and wilt do that which is right in his sight, and wilt give ear to his commandments, and keep all his statutes, I will put none of these diseases upon thee, which I have brought upon the Egyptians: for I am the LORD that healeth thee.* (The Hebrew word used here is *Jehovah-Rapha*.)

## God Heals Because His Enemy Makes People Sick.

Jesus came to destroy the works of the devil (adversary).

*I John 3:8* - *He that committeth sin is of the devil; for the devil sinneth from the beginning. For this purpose the Son of God was manifested, that he might destroy the works of the devil.*

*Matt 12:15* - *But when Jesus knew it, he withdrew himself from thence: and great multitudes followed him, and he healed them all.*

*Luke 6:17-19* – *And he came down with them, and stood in the plain, and the company of his disciples, and a great multitude of people out of all Judaea and Jerusalem, and from the sea coast of Tyre and Sidon, which came to hear him. and to be healed of their diseases; 18. And they that were vexed with unclean spirits: and they were healed. 19. And the whole multitude sought to touch him: for there went virtue out of him, and healed them all.*

*Acts 10:38* - *How God anointed Jesus of Nazareth with the Holy Ghost and with power: who went about doing good, and healing all that were oppressed of the devil; for God was with him.*

In all these verses Jesus is shown to healing, saving, delivering, setting free, and unloosing people from every type of physical, mental, and spiritual hindrance regardless of how small or large.

Now let's look at a case in point.

***Luke 13:10-17*** *– And he was teaching in one of the synagogues on the Sabbath. 11. And, behold, there was a woman which had a spirit of infirmity eighteen years, and was bowed together, and could in no wise lift up herself.*

(This woman had been in this condition for eighteen years, most likely coming to the synagogue regularly, yet those in leadership had never helped her.)

*Vs 12. And when Jesus saw her, he called her to him, and said unto her, Woman, thou art loosed from thine infirmity.*

(Jesus told the woman she was loosed while she was still bowed over. This is preaching (proclaiming) deliverance to the captives.)

*Vs 13. And he laid his hands on her: and immediately she was made straight, and glorified God.* (Jesus spoke and then acted He did not just teach. He demonstrated the gospel. A gospel (good news) that is not demonstrated is not good news but rather cruel teasing.) *14. And the ruler of the synagogue answered with indignation, because that Jesus had healed on the Sabbath day, and said unto the people, There are six days in which men ought to work: in them therefore come and be healed, and not on the Sabbath day.*

(This is always the reaction of a religious spirit. Notice that they did not argue over whether or not Jesus could heal or would heal, which would have been useless since Jesus was doing it right in front of them. The religious spirit will always condemn you for doing what they know they should be doing, but aren't. Usually their tactic involves condemning the way you are doing it more than whether or not you should be doing it. They were saying that there were other days in which to heal, yet they were not doing on any day.)

*Vs. 15. The Lord then answered him, and said, Thou hypocrite, doth not each one of you on the Sabbath loose his ox or his ass from the stall, and lead him away to watering?*

(This shows God's viewpoint of acting one way in day to day affairs and another in religious affairs. Anyone that separates their life into a "real life" category and a "church" category is a hypocrite. Anyone that does more for an animal than they would or do for a human is a hypocrite.)

Vs *16. And ought not this woman, being a daughter of Abraham whom Satan hath bound, lo, these eighteen years, be loosed from this bond on the Sabbath day?*

(The only reason Jesus gave for the woman's healing was the fact that she was a daughter of Abraham. Paul said that the true children of Abraham were those that were Jews in the heart and not by the flesh. He went on to say that anyone of faith was a Jew. Since this is the only reason Jesus gave, it should he enough for anyone. We also see that she had been bound for 18 years and that; Jesus said that Satan had bound her for 18 years. He also proved that no day should be too special for a child of God to minister healing or be healed.)

Vs *17. And when he had said these things, all his adversaries were ashamed: and all the people rejoiced for all the glorious things that were done by him.*

(This will always he the result of faith and healing, God's adversaries will he ashamed and the people will rejoice and glorify God)

**God Heals Because Jesus Paid For Mankind's Healing.**

You are not your own - you are bought with a price.

*I Corinthians 6:19-20* – *What? know ye not that your body is the temple of the Holy Ghost which is in you, which ye have of God, and ye are not your own? 20. For ye are bought with a price: therefore glorify God in your body, and in your spirit, which are God's.*

Jesus suffered your sickness so you would not have to.

*Malt 8:17* - *That it might be fulfilled which was spoken by Esaias the prophet, saying, Himself took our infirmities, and bare our sicknesses.*

*1 Peter 2:24* - *Who his own self bare our sins in his own body on the tree, that we, being dead to sins, should live unto righteousness: by whose stripes ye were healed.*

Healing is in the atonement - (See above) Matt. 8:17 / 1 Pet. 2:24

Your body is the Temple of the Holy Ghost. (1 Corinthians 6:19)

If sickness in the Old Testament made people "unclean" why would the Holy Ghost want to reside in a polluted body?

You are the church which is the body of Christ. *Ephesians 1:22-23 – And hath put all things under his feet, and gave him to be the head over all things to the church, Which is his body, the fulness of him that filleth all in all.*

Did Jesus plan on having a disabled, sick, diseased body?

Under the Old Covenant a person was not even eligible to be a priest unless their body was without defect.

**God Heals because healing, salvation, and deliverance are all the same to Him.**

To God there is no difference in the size of the need. He does not have to exert Himself anymore to heal than to save. Man is the only creature than categorizes things in this manner. God has not differentiated between the two. The devil, the enemy of God and man is the originator of the idea that we must decide between the two or be satisfied with salvation from sin. The very word used in the Bible for salvation means health, healing, deliverance, prosperity, peace, and wholeness. Salvation is the all-inclusive word in the Bible which clearly defines Gods attitude and will for us. In the absolute truest sense of the meaning of the word "salvation", we cannot say that we are truly and totally "saved" unless all of the above definition can be applied to every area of our life. If you have accepted Jesus as your Lord and Savior but remain in sickness, you cannot claim to be "saved to the uttermost", this does not mean that if you died or if Jesus returned that you would not go to Heaven. It just means that there is more of the blood of Jesus that can be applied to areas in your life. By the same token, if you are healed of a disease but have not made Jesus your Lord, you are not totally saved either. Here's another way to look at this: A man with a terminal disease was drowning in a river and a person came along and pulled them out. We could say that the drowning man was "saved", yet he still has the terminal disease and will die unless something happens. The man that pulled the drowning man from the river is a "savior" in a limited way. But what if the man with the terminal disease was pulled from the river by a doctor that knew the cure for the terminal disease?

Now the man that pulled the drowning man from the river is his "savior" in a wider capacity. This is obviously a picture of God and man. God can be your limited Savior or He can be your complete Savior. We must not limit God in our lives. We must remember what happened to those who limited God in the Old Testament.

*Psalm 78:1-72* - *Give ear, 0 my people, to my law: incline your ears to the words of my mouth. 2 I will open my mouth in a parable: I will utter dark sayings of old: 3 Which we have heard and known, and our fathers have told us. 4. We will not hide them from their children, shewing to the generation to come the praises of the LORD, and his strength, and his wonderful works that he hath done. 5. For he established a testimony in Jacob, and appointed a law in Israel, which he commanded our fathers, that they should make them known to their children: 6. That the generation to come might know them, even the children which should be born; who should arise and declare them to their children: 7. That they might set their hope in God and not forget the works of God but keep his commandments: 8. And might not be as their fathers, a stubborn and rebellious generation; a generation that set not their heart aright, and whose spirit was not stedfast with God. 9. The children of Ephraim, being armed and carrying bows, turned back in the* day of battle. 10. They kept not the covenant of God, and refused to walk in his law; 11. And forgat his works, and his wonders that he had shewed them. 12. Marvellous things did he in the sight of their fathers, in the land of Egypt, in the field of Zoan. 13. He divided the sea, and caused them to pass through; and he made the waters to stand as an heap. 14. In the daytime also he led them with a cloud, and all the night with a light of fire. 15. He clave the rocks in the wilderness, and gave them drink as out of the great depths. 16. He brought streams also out of the rock, and caused waters to run down like rivers. 17. And they sinned yet more against him by provoking the most High in the wilderness. 18. And they tempted God in their heart by asking meat for their lust. 19 Yea, they spake against God; they said, Can God furnish a table in the wilderness? 20. Behold, he smote the rock, that the waters gushed out, and the streams overflowed; can he give bread also? can he provide flesh for his people? 21. Therefore the LORD heard this, and was wroth: so a fire was kindled against Jacob, and anger also came up against Israel; 22. Because they believed not in God, and trusted not in his salvation: 23. Though he had commanded the clouds from above, and opened the doors of heaven, 24. And had rained down manna upon them to eat, and had given them of the corn of heaven. 25 Man did eat angels' food: he sent them meat to the full. 26. He caused an east wind to blow in the heaven: and by his power he brought in the south wind. 27. He rained flesh also upon them as dust, and feathered fowls like as the sand of the sea: 28. And he let it fall in the midst of their camp, round about their habitations. 29. So they did eat, and were well filled: for he gave them their own desire; 30. They were not estranged from their lust. But while their meat was yet in their mouths, 31. The wrath of God came upon them, and slew the fattest of them, and smote down the chosen men of Israel. 32. For all this they sinned still, and believed not for his wondrous works. 33. Therefore their days did he consume in vanity, and their years in trouble. 34. When he slew them, then they sought him: and they returned and inquired early after God. 35. And they remembered that God was their rock, and the high God their redeemer. 36. Nevertheless they did flatter him with their mouth and they lied unto him with their tongues. 37. For their heart was not right with him, neither were they stedfast in his covenant 38.But he, being full of compassion, forgave their iniquity, and destroyed them not: yea, many at time turned he his anger away, and did not stir up all his wrath. 39. For he remembered that they were but flesh; a wind that passeth away, and cometh not again. 40. How oft did they provoke him in the wilderness, and grieve him in the desert! 41. Yea they turned back and tempted God and limited the Holy One of

Israel. 42. They remembered not his hand, nor the day when he delivered them from the enemy. 43. How he had wrought his signs in Egypt, and his wonders in the field of Zoan: 44. And had turned their rivers into blood; and their floods, that they could not drink. 45. He sent divers sorts of flies among them, which devoured them; and frogs, which destroyed them. 46. He gave also their increase unto the caterpillar, and their labour unto the locust. 47. He destroyed their vines with hail, and their sycamore trees with frost 48. He gave up their cattle also to the hail, and their flocks to hot thunderbolts. 49. He cast upon them the fierceness of his anger, wrath, and indignation, and trouble, by sending evil angels among them. 50. He made a way to his anger, he spared not their soul from death, but gave their life over to the pestilence; 51. And smote all the firstborn in Egypt; the chief of their strength in the tabernacles of Ham: 52. But made his own people to go forth like sheep, and guided them in the wilderness like a flock. 53. And he led them on safely, so that they feared not: but the sea overwhelmed their enemies. 54. And he brought them to the border of his sanctuary, even to this mountain, which his right hand had purchased. 55. He cast out the heathen also before them, and divided them an inheritance by line, and made the tribes of Israel to dwell in their tents. 56. Yet they tempted and provoked the most high God and kept not his testimonies: 57. But turned back and dealt *unfaithfully like their fathers: they were turned aside like a deceitful bow. 58. For they provoked him to anger with their high places and moved him to jealousy with their graven images. 59. When God heard this, he was wroth, and greatly abhorred Israel: 60. So that he forsook the tabernacle of Shiloh, the tent which he placed among men; 61. And delivered his strength into captivity, and his glory into the enemy's hand. 62. He gave his people over also unto the sword; and was wroth with his inheritance. 63. The fire consumed their young men; and their maidens were not given to marriage. 64. Their priests fell by the sword; and their widows made no lamentation. 65. Then the Lord awaked as one out of sleep, and like a mighty man that shouteth by reason of wine. 66. And he smote his enemies in the hinder parts: he put them to a perpetual reproach. 67. Moreover he refused the tabernacle of Joseph, and chose not the tribe of Ephraim: 68. But chose the tribe of Judith, the mount Zion which he loved. 69. And he built his sanctuary like high palaces, like the earth which he hath established for ever. 70. He chose David also his servant, and took him from the sheepfolds: 71. From following the ewes great with young he brought him to feed Jacob his people, and Israel his inheritance. 72. So he fed them according to the integrity of his heart, and guided them by the skilfulness of his hands.*

You can see by this Psalm that God expects those to whom and through whom He shows His power, to stay close to Him, to tell of His wondrous works, to pass on their faith to their children. The Hebrews tempted and provoked God by limiting Him. If we are under a better covenant, how much more should we remember His works? Do not limit God. Is there anything to hard for Him?

**Scriptural Reasons God Heals.**

*Psalm 91:14-16* - *Because he hath set his love upon me therefore will I deliver him: I will set him on high, because he hath known my name. 15. He shall call upon me, and I will answer him: I will be with him in trouble; I will deliver him, and honour ham 16. With long life will I satisfy him and shew him my salvation.*

In Deuteronomy 28 we are told what will happen if we obey God and what will happen if we disobey God. Healing of every sickness and disease is under the blessings listed if we obey God and those same sicknesses and diseases are listed as the curse that shall come upon us if we do not obey God. If you have sinned and became sick or diseased, it is an easy thing to repent, receive forgiveness and be healed.

If you are converted, you should be healed.

**Matt 13:14-15** – *And in them is fulfilled the prophecy of Esaias, which saith, By hearing ye shall hear, and shall not understand; and seeing ye shall see, and shall not perceive: 15. For this people's heart is waxed gross, and their ears are dull of hearing, and their eyes they have closed; lest at any time they should see with their eyes, and hear with their ears, and should understand with their heart, and should be converted, and I should heal them.*

**Psalm 103:1-6** - *Bless the LORD, 0 my soul: and all that is within me, bless his holy name. 2 Bless the LORD, 0 my soul, and forget not all his benefits: 3. Who forgiveth all thine iniquities; who healeth all thy diseases; 4. Who redeemeth thy life from destruction; who crowned' thee with lovingkindness and tender mercies; 5. Who satisfieth thy mouth with good things; so that thy youth is renewed like the eagle's. 6. The LORD executeth righteousness and judgment for all that are oppressed.*

(We are commanded not to forget ALL His benefits. Yet that is what we do. These are His benefits - He forgives All our sin and sins AND HE HEALS All our diseases. These are the

143

two compartments that man must deal with in this life - the spiritual and the physical. If what was just said did not clear it up God then reiterates by saying that He redeems our life from destruction and He crowns us with lovingkindness and tender mercies, not sickness and crippling afflictions. If you will look at most of the healings Jesus performed you will find that they were performed in answer to a cry for MERCY. In verse 6 we are told that the Lord executes righteousness and judgment for (or in favor of) everyone that is oppressed This does not mean that God is the one judging the oppressed because that would not be in keeping with the spirit of what is being written in this passage of scripture. It is obviously saying that God judges in favor of the oppressed meaning that He judges righteously when He declares that the oppressed are to be freed. We are also told in Psalm 34:19 - Many are the afflictions of the righteous: but the LORD delivereth him out of them all.

☐

# Chapter 5:

## Where Does God Heal?

### I. Bible Places God Has Healed People.

#### In Church - Synagogue.

*Mark 1:21-28* – And they went into Capernaum; and straightway on the Sabbath day he entered into the synagogue, and taught. 22. And they were astonished at his doctrine: for he taught them as one that had authority, and not as the scribes. 23. And there was in their synagogue a man with an unclean spirit and he cried out 24. Saying, Let us alone; what have we to do with thee, thou Jesus of Nazareth? Art thou come to destroy us? I know thee who thou art, the Holy One of God. 25. And Jesus rebuked him saying Hold thy peace, and come out of him. 26. And when the unclean spirit had torn him and cried with a loud voice, he came out of him. 27. And they were all amazed, insomuch that they questioned among themselves, saying, what thing is this? What new doctrine is this? For with authority commanded' he even the unclean spirits, and they do obey him. 28. And immediately his fame spread abroad throughout all the region round about Galilee.

**In the Market Place and in the public streets.**

*Mark 1:32-34* – And at even, when the sun did set, they brought unto him all that were diseased, and them that were possessed with devils. 33. And all the city was gathered together at the door. 34. And he healed many that were sick of divers diseases, and cast out many devils; and suffered not the devils to speak, because they knew him.

*Acts 14:8-11* – And there sat a certain man at Lystra. impotent in his feet, being a cripple from his mother's womb, who never had walked: 9. The same heard Paul speak: who stedfastly beholding him, and perceiving that he had faith to be healed, 10. Said with a loud voice, Stand upright on thy feet. And he leaped and walked. 11. And when the people saw what Paul had done, they lifted up their voices, saying in the speech of Lycaonia, the gods are come down to us in the likeness of men.

*Acts 5:12-16* – And by the hands of the apostles were many signs and wonders wrought among the people; (and they
146

were all with one accord in Solomon's porch. 13. And of the rest durst no man join himself to them: but the people magnified them. 14. And believers were the more added to the Lord, multitudes both of men and women.) 15. Insomuch that they brought forth the sick into the streets, and laid them on beds and couches, that at the least the shadow of Peter passing by might overshadow some of them. 16. There came also a multitude out of the cities round about unto Jerusalem, bringing sick folks, and them which were vexed with unclean spirits: and they were healed every one.

**Mark 10:46-52** – And they came to Jericho: and as he went out of Jericho with his disciples and a great number of people, blind Bartimaeus, the son of Timaeus, sat by the highway side begging. 47. And when he heard that it was Jesus of Nazareth, he began to cry out, and say, Jesus, thou Son of David, have mercy on me. 48. And many charged him that he should hold his peace: but he cried the more a great deal, Thou Son of David, have mercy on me. 49. And Jesus stood still, and commanded him to be called. And they call the blind man, saying unto him, be of good comfort, rise; he calleth thee. 50. And he, casting away his garment, rose, and came to Jesus. 51. And Jesus answered and said unto him, What wilt thou that I should do unto thee? The blind man said unto him, Lord, that I might receive my sight. 52. And Jesus said unto him, Go thy way; thy faith hath made thee whole. And immediately he received his sight, and followed Jesus in the way.

## In Homes:

### In Jewish homes.

*Matt 8:14-15* – And when Jesus was come into Peter's house, he saw his wife's mother laid, and sick of a fever. 15. And he touched her hand, and the fever left her: and she arose, and ministered unto them.

*Acts 20:7-12* – And upon the first day of the week, when the disciples came together to break bread, Paul preached unto them, ready to depart on the morrow; and continued his speech until midnight. 8. And there were many lights in the upper chamber where they were gathered together. 9. And there sat in a window a certain young man named Eutychus, being fallen into a deep sleep: and as Paul was long preaching, he sunk down with sleep, and fell down from the third loft and was taken up dead. 10 And Paul went down, and fell on him, and embracing him said, Trouble not yourselves; for his life is in him. 11. When he therefore was come up again, and had broken bread, and eaten, and talked a long while, even till break of day, so he departed. 12. And they brought the young man alive, and were not a little comforted.

**Mark 1:29-31** – And forthwith, when they were come out of the synagogue, they entered into the house of Simon and Andrew with James and John. 30. But Simon's wife's mother lay sick of a fever, and anon they tell him of her. 31. And he came and took her by the hand, and lifted her up; and immediately the fever left her, and she ministered unto them.

**In Gentile homes**.

**Matt 8:5-13** -- And when Jesus was entered into Capernaum, there came unto him a centurion,. (A gentile) beseeching him, 6. And saying, Lord, my servant lieth at home sick of the palsy, grievously tormented. 7. And Jesus saith unto him I will come and heal him. 8. The centurion answered and said, Lord, I am not worthy that thou shouldest come under my roof: but speak the word only, and my servant shall be healed. 9. For I am a man under authority, having soldiers under me: and I say to this man, Go, and he goeth; and to another, Come, and he corneth; and to my servant, Do this, and he doeth it. 10. When Jesus heard it, he marveled, and said to them that followed, *Verily I say unto you, I have not found so great faith, no, not in Israel. 11. And I say unto you, that many shall come from the east and west, and shall sit down with Abraham, and Isaac, and Jacob, in the kingdom of heaven. 12. But the children of the kingdom shall be east out into outer darkness: there shall be weeping and gnashing of teeth. 13. And Jesus said unto the centurion, Go thy way; and as thou hast believed, so be it done unto thee. And his servant was healed in the selfsame hour.*

**In the Desert.** (The Israelites)

For 40 years they were either kept healthy or healed.

2. **Numbers 21:7-9** – *Therefore the people came to Moses, and said, We have sinned, for we have spoken against the LORD, and against thee; pray unto the LORD, that he take away the serpents from us. And Moses prayed for the people. 8. And the LORD said unto Moses, Make thee a fiery serpent, and set it upon a pole: and it shall come to pass, that every one that is bitten, when he looketh upon it, shall Live. 9. And Moses made a serpent of brass, and put it upon a pole, and it came to pass, that if a serpent had bitten any man, when he beheld the serpent of brass, he lived.*

150

In Bondage. (The Israelites being set free)

Not one feeble among their numbers.

**Psalm 107:37** - *He brought them forth also with silver and gold: and there was not one feeble person among their tribes.*

The Hebrew word *kashal* (kaw-shal'); translated here as "feeble" is # 3782 in the Strong's Concordance and means: to totter or waver (through weakness of the legs, especially the ankle); by implication, to falter, stumble, faint or fall. Obviously they (the Hebrews) were not a sick, diseased bunch of people. The idea that there would not be even 1 person sick or diseased or "weak and tottering" in a nation of 1 to 3 million people, is obviously not very realistic. Anyone that had been sick, was apparently healed as they partook of the passover meal the night before they left their bondage. The Passover Meal was actually the beginning or initiation of their freedom. Again, we have a type of the Christian life with the Communion or Lord's Supper symbolizing and celebrating our freedom from sin and sickness. Just as we commemorate the forgiveness of our sins when we partake of the cup/blood, we should also receive healing as we partake of the bread/body "which was broken for you".

In distant places. See Point 2.a. (Matt. 8:5) above.

☐

# Chapter 6:

## How Does God Heal?

**I. Scriptural methods God has used to Heal.**

**The Spoken Word.**

***Matt 9:2-7*** *– And, behold, they brought to him a man sick of the palsy, lying on a bed: and Jesus seeing their faith said unto the sick of the palsy; Son, be of good cheer; thy sins be forgiven thee. 3. And, behold, certain of the scribes said within themselves, This man blasphemeth. 4. And Jesus knowing their thoughts said, Wherefore think ye evil in your hearts? 5. For whether is easier, to say, Thy sins be forgiven thee; or to say, Arise, and walk? 6. But that ye may know that the Son of man hath power on earth to forgive sins, (then saith he to the sick of the palsy,) Arise, take up thy bed, and go unto thine house. 7 And he arose, and departed to his house.*

## Anointed Prayer Cloths.

*Acts 19:11-12* – *And God wrought special miracles by the hands of Paul: 12. So that from his body were brought unto the sick handkerchiefs or aprons, and the diseases departed from them, and the evil spirits went out of them.*

*Matt 9:20-22* – *And, behold, a woman, which was diseased with an issue of blood twelve years, came behind him, and touched the hem of his garment: 21. For she said within herself, If I may but touch his garment, I shall be whole. 22. But Jesus turned him about, and when he saw her, He said, Daughter, be of good comfort; thy faith had made thee whole. And the woman was made whole from that hour.*

## Dipping in the Jordan River 7 Times.

*II Kings 5:10 & 14* –*(10) And Elisha sent a messenger unto him, saying, Go and wash in Jordan seven times, and thy flesh shall come again to thee, and thou shalt be clean.*

*(14) Then went he down, and dipped himself seven times in Jordan, according to the saying of the man of God: and his flesh came again like unto the flesh of a little child, and he was clean. (KJV)*

**Spit & Mud**.

*John 9:5-7* - *As long as I am in the world, I am the light of the world. 6 When he had thus spoken, he spat on the ground, and made clay of the spittle, and he anointed the eyes of the blind man with the clay, 7 And said unto him, Go, wash in the pool of Siloam, (which is by interpretation, Sent.) He went his way therefore, and washed, and came seeing.*

**Laying on of Hands.**

*Matt 19:15* - *And he laid his hands on them, and departed thence.*

*Mark 6:5* - *And he could there do no mighty work, save that he laid his hands upon a few sick folk, and healed them.*

*Luke 4:40* - *Now when the sun was setting, all they that had any sick with divers diseases brought them unto him; and He laid his hands on every one of them, and healed them*

*Luke 13:13* - *And he laid his hands on her: and immediately she was made straight, and glorified God.*

*Acts 19:6* - *And when Paul had laid his hands upon them, the Holy Ghost came on them; and they spake with tongues, and prophesied.*

*Acts 28:8* - *And it came to pass, that the father of Publius lay sick of a fever and of a bloody flux: to whom Paul entered in, and prayed, and laid his hands on him., and healed him.*

## Praying for One Another.

*James 5:16* - *Confess your faults one to another, and pray one for another, that ye may be healed. The effectual fervent prayer of a righteous man availeth much.*

## The Prayer of Faith.

**James 5:15** - And the prayer of faith shall save the sick, and the Lord shall raise him up; and if he have committed sins, they shall be forgiven him.

## Anointing With Oil.

*James 5:14* - *is any sick among you? Let him call for the elders of the church; and let them pray over him, anointing him with oil in the name of the Lord:*

*Mark 6:13* - *And they cast out many devils, and anointed with oil many that were sick, and healed them.*

## Asking and Receiving

*Matt 7:7* - *Ask, and it shall be given you; seek, and ye shall find; knock, and it shall be opened unto you:*

*Matt 18:19* - *Again I say unto you, That if two of you shall agree on earth as touching any thing that they shall ask, it shall be done for them of my Father which is in heaven.*

*Matt 21:22* - *And all things, whatsoever ye shall ask in prayer, believing, ye shall receive.*

*Luke 11:9-10* -*9 And I say unto you, Ask, and it shall be given you; seek, and ye shall find; knock, and it shall be opened unto you. 10 For every one that asketh receiveth; and* he that seeketh findeth; and to him that knocketh it shall be opened.

*John 14:13* - And whatsoever ye shall ask in my name, that will I do, that the Father may be glorified in the Son.

*John 14:14* - If ye shall ask any thing in my name, I will do it.

*John 15:7* - If ye abide in me, and my words abide in you, ye shall ask what ye will, and it shall be done unto you.

*John 15:16* - Ye have not chosen me, but I have chosen you, and ordained you, that ye should go and bring forth fruit, and that your fruit should remain: that whatsoever ye shall ask of the Father in my name, he may give it you.

*John 16:24* - Hitherto have ye asked nothing in my name: ask, and ye shall receive, that your joy may be full.

*John 16:26* - At that day ye shall ask in my name: and I say not unto you, that I will pray the Father for you:

*James 1:6* - *But let him ask in faith, nothing wavering. For he that wavereth is like a wave of the sea driven with the wind and tossed.*

*James 4:2* - *Ye lust, and have not: ye kill, and desire to have, and cannot obtain: ye fight and war, yet ye have not, because ye ask not.*

*1 John 5:14* - *And this is the confidence that we have in him, that, if we ask any thing according to his will, he heareth us:*

*1 John 5:15* - *And if we know that he hear us, whatsoever we ask, we know that we have the petitions that we desired of him.*

**Point of Contact –**

Touching the hem of Jesus' Garment.
(See point 2. b. Matt. 9:20-22 above)

**Through Communion.**

*1 Cor. 11:28-31* - *28 But let a man examine himself, and so let him eat of that bread, and drink of that cup. 29 For he that eateth and drinketh unworthily, eateth and drinketh damnation to himself, not discerning the Lord's body. 30 For this cause many are weak and sickly among you, and many sleep. 31 For if we would judge ourselves, we should not be judged.*

*I Cor. 11:24* - *And when he had given thanks, he brake it, and said, Take, eat: this is my body, which is broken for you: this do in remembrance of me.*

*Luke 22:19* - *And he took bread, and gave thanks, and brake it, and gave unto them, saying, This is my body which is given for you: this do in remembrance of me.*

*Mark 14:22-24* – *And as they did eat, Jesus took bread, and blessed, and brake it, and gave to them, and said, Take, eat: this is my body. 23. And he took the cup, and when he had given thanks, he gave it to them: and they all drank of it. 24. And he said unto them, This is my blood of the new testament, which is shed for many.*

Looking unto the Brazen Serpent.

*Numbers 21:8-9 – And the LORD said unto Moses, Make thee a fiery serpent, and set it upon a pole: and it shall come to pass, that every one that is bitten, when he looketh upon it, shall live. 9. And Moses made a serpent of brass, and put it upon a pole, and it came to pass, that if a serpent had bitten any man, when he beheld the serpent of brass, he lived.*

# Chapter 7:

## What Are You Going To Do Now?

### Summary

It should be obvious to you by now that God will heal anyone, anywhere, anytime, of anything. He has healed sinners, saints, kings, peasants, men, women, children, prophets, pagans, and even those who were killing His people and persecuting the church. There is literally no one beyond God's healing reach. The only prerequisite for healing has been and always will be faith. This is where some lose heart because they have been told that they must have faith. While this may be a common teaching today, it is not true. All that is required is that someone have faith. If the sick person does not have faith then it becomes the duty of the believer to believe (have faith) for them.

The hardest people to get healed is usually Christians because they feel that they have failed to live up to the Bible standard for the Christian, (which is true, because if we could live up to the standard on our own, Christ would not have had

163

to die for us), so now they feel unworthy for God to heal them or they feel as though they must do something to make up for their wrongs and therefore become good enough to be healed. This is the trap Satan sets, first to tempt you to sin, then to condemn you for sinning so that you are unable to go to God and receive His forgiveness, if you do get that far, he will still continually keep you beat down by the weight and guilt of the fact that you sinned which keeps you ineffective in the Kingdom of God. Remember, the size of the gift from the Giver does not depend upon the goodness of the messenger or the worthiness of the receiver. Just believe that God is bigger than your sin and receive the free gift of healing just as you did salvation. The same goes for the one ministering healing. Just keep laying hands on people and praying the prayer of faith, regardless of what you are going through. If God could only use perfect people to work through He would never get anything done. He uses what has been made AVAILABLE to Him.

**Take Heed to what you hear.**

*Mark 4:24-29 – And he said unto them, Take heed what ye hear: with what measure ye mete, it shall be measured to you: and unto you that hear shall more be given. 25. For he that hath, to him shall be given: and he that hath not, from him shall* be taken even that which he hath. 26. And he said, So is the kingdom of God, as if a man should cast seed into the ground; 27. And should sleep, and rise night and day, and the seed should spring and grow up, he knoweth not how. 28. For the earth bringeth forth fruit of herself; first the blade, then the ear, after that the full corn in the ear. 29. But when the fruit is brought forth, immediately he putteth in the sickle, because the harvest is come.

**He that heareth My Sayings and doeth them not is a fool.**

*Luke 6:47-49* – Whosoever cometh to me, and heareth my sayings, and doeth them, I will shew you to whom he is like: 48. He is like a man which built an house, and digged deep, and laid the foundation on a rock: and when the flood arose, the stream beat vehemently upon that house, and could not shake it: for it was founded upon a rock. 49. But he that heareth, and doeth not, is like a man that without a foundation built an house upon the earth; against which the stream did beat vehemently, and immediately it fell; and the ruin of that house was great.

**To Whom Much is given, much is required.**

*Luke 12:42-48 – And the Lord said, Who then is that faithful and wise steward, whom his lord shall make ruler over his household, to give them their portion of meat in due season? 43. Blessed is that servant, whom his lord when he cometh shall find so doing. 44. Of a truth I say unto you, that he will make him ruler over all that he hath. 45. But and if that servant say in his heart, My lord delayeth his coming; and shall begin to beat the menservants and maidens, and to eat and drink, and to be drunken; 46. The lord of that servant will come in a day when he looketh not for him, and at an hour when he is not aware, and will cut him in sunder, and will appoint him his portion with the unbelievers. 47. And that servant, which knew his lord's will, and prepared not himself, neither did according to his will, shall be beaten with many stripes. 48. But he that knew not, and did commit things worthy of stripes, shall be beaten with few stripes. For unto whomsoever much is given, of him shall be much required: and to whom men have committed much, of him they will ask the more.*

**He that knows to do good and doeth it not it is sin.**

*James 4:17* - *Therefore to him that knoweth to do good, and doeth it not, to him it is sin.*

**Jesus went about doing good and healing all...**

*Acts 10:38* - *How God anointed Jesus of Nazareth with the Holy Ghost and with power: who went about doing good, and healing all that were oppressed of the devil; for God was with him.* (KJV)

**Walk in the light you have.**

*Luke 12:48* - *But he that knew not, and did commit things worthy of stripes, shall be beaten with few stripes. For unto whomsoever much is given, of him shall be much required: and to whom men have committed much, of him they will ask the more.*

**The Golden Rule.**

*Matthew 7:12* - *Therefore all things whatsoever ye would that men should do to you, do ye even so to them: for this is the law and the prophets.*

(This tells us that if we were sick and we knew of someone that had the power of God to heal the sick (aka: The Baptism of the Holy Spirit) and we would want them to come to us, then we are morally obligated to go to them and pray the prayer of faith and get them healed.)

## About the Author

Dr. Larry L Yates is a Minister, Author and Bible Teacher. He is President and Co-founder, with his wife Shelia of Mineola Bible Institute, an Apostolic teaching ministry dedicated to sharing the Apostolic Faith, the revelation of our Full Salvation and the realities of the New Creation to lost and hurting humanity through advanced understanding of the truth and reality of God's Word.

He graduated in 1985 with a degree in Professional Nursing and is a retired Trauma Nurse/Paramedic. Larry holds a Master's Degree in Theology from Apostolic Theological Bible College in Tampa, Florida and graduated *summa cum laude* with dual Doctorates in Theology and Religion from Cypress Bible Institute and Calvary Bible College and Seminary. He completed his Doctor of Ministry at Great Commission Bible College in Kiefer, OK.

He is the author of *"The Divided God: Apostolic Theology and the Biblical Challenge to Contemporary Trinitarianism,"* as well as *"Releasing the Anointing: How to Pray an Hour Without Repeating Yourself."*

Larry is President of Miracles in Action as well as a faculty member and member of the Board of Regents of the International Apostolic University, in the UK. In addition, he is affiliated with the International Apostolic Council, in Dallas, TX.

He lives in Mineola, Texas with his wife and daughter. Their mission is to boldly and fearlessly proclaim the Apostolic Message, without compromise, everywhere they go. Larry has a unique ability to empathize with those who hunger for spiritual reality rather than the bondage of religion and the traditions of men. His "Back to the Basics" approach is simple, yet profoundly effective as he teaches believers the truths of God while helping them to understand who they are in Christ.

Larry may be contacted for ministry or information at:

**drlarrylyates@gmail.com**

**www.mineolabibleinstitute.org**